THE FORCE
of
BEAUTY

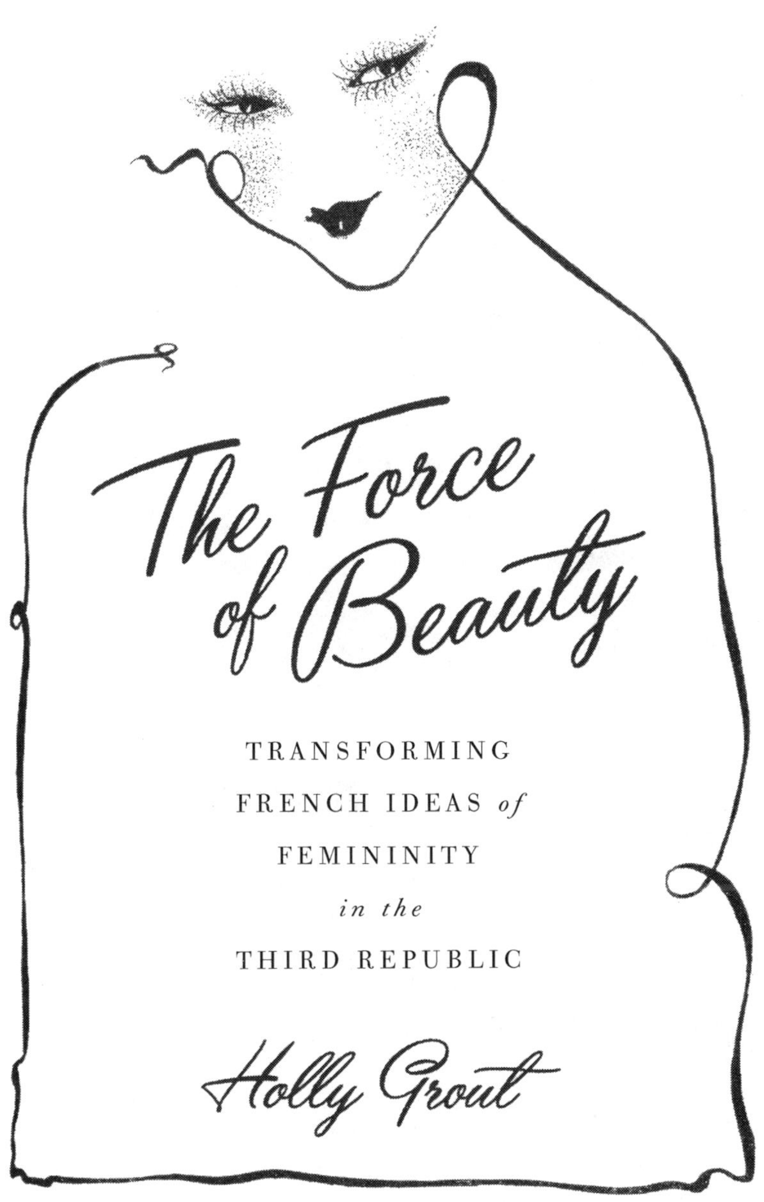

The Force of Beauty

TRANSFORMING
FRENCH IDEAS *of*
FEMININITY
in the
THIRD REPUBLIC

Holly Grout

Louisiana State University Press Baton Rouge

Published by Louisiana State University Press

Manufactured in the United States of America
First printing

Designer: Michelle A. Neustrom
Typeface: Corda
Printer and binder: Maple Press

Library of Congress Cataloging-in-Publication Data
Grout, Holly, 1976–
The force of beauty : transforming French ideas of femininity in the Third Republic / Holly Grout.
pages cm
Includes bibliographical references and index.
ISBN 978-0-8071-5988-0 (cloth : alk. paper) — ISBN 978-0-8071-5989-7 (pdf) — ISBN 978-0-8071-5990-3 (epub) — ISBN 978-0-8071-5991-0 (mobi) 1. Aesthetics—Social aspects—History. 2. Beauty, Personal—France—History. 3. Femininity—France—History. 4. Women—France—Social conditions. 5. France—Social life and customs. 6. France—History—Third Republic, 1870–1940. I. Title.
HQ1220.F8G76 2015
305.40944—dc23

2014038673

The paper in this book meets the guidelines for permanence and durability of the Committee on Production Guidelines for Book Longevity of the Council on Library Resources. ♾

Contents

Acknowledgments

I am profoundly grateful to colleagues, friends, and family, without whom *The Force of Beauty* would not have been realized. My greatest debt is to Laird Boswell and Mary Louise Roberts, the best of all possible advisors, who patiently guided me through this project from its inception. Laird valiantly weathered my "nutty theories," and his meticulous readings of my work have made me a better researcher, a better writer, and a better scholar. Lou has challenged me, from dissertation draft to manuscript revision, to ask the difficult questions, to trust my instincts, and to recognize the broader implications of my work. Lou's and Laird's generosity with their time and with their praise, their intellectual rigor, and their devotion to the project of learning have influenced me beyond measure. My greatest appreciation as well to teachers and scholars Suzanne Desan, Rudy Koshar, Ellen Furlough, Jeremy Popkin, and Whitney Walton, who taught by example that integrity is necessary in scholarship as well as within the scholar.

Grants and fellowships provided by the Institut d'études politiques de Paris, the University of Wisconsin-Madison, the American Institute for the History of Pharmacy, and the University of Alabama made the research for this book financially possible. This book would not have been possible without the resources of several libraries and archives, including the Bibliothèque nationale de France, the Bibliothèque Forney, the Bibliothèque Marguerite Durand, the Bibliothèque historique de la Ville de Paris, the Archives nationales de France, and the Archives de Paris. Thanks to my editor, Alisa Plant, for believing in this project and for helping me bring it to fruition.

Numerous colleagues and friends have patiently listened to my musings, graciously read and commented on chapters, and critically engaged the project at every stage. In Paris, Rachel Nuñez and I spent (perhaps too many!) long hours together in the BN indulgently discussing nineteenth-century French women, while I benefitted immensely from the research tips, translation advice, and friendship proffered by Adeline Bertheault, Rob Lewis, Nick Toloudis, and Rebecca Scales. Ethan Katz, Hunter Martin, Bill Meier, Kendra Smith-Howard, Nicholas Wolf, and members of the Wisconsin French History Group provided invaluable feedback on early versions of the work. At Alabama, I have found charitable colleagues, judicious readers, and kind friends in Margaret Abruzzo, Steve Bunker, Andrew Huebner, Heather Kopelson, Jimmy Mixson, Dan Riches, and members of the Eurohist workshop. Thanks as well to the students who have taught me so much and who continue to inspire me.

This project would not have reached completion, nor would I have maintained my sanity through it, without the fabulous Sunday morning Edelweiss writing club. My deepest gratitude to Dan Sweaney and honorary member Matt Orndorff, who have provided countless hours of fun and laughter; to Jolene Hubbs and Sarah Moody, who encourage me to work harder, to laugh louder, and to be kinder to myself; and to Jenny Shaw, who enthusiastically read and reread version after version of so many bits and pieces of chapters, proposals, and conference papers, who continues to act as sounding board and coconspirator, and without whom I would have far less confidence.

I am also grateful for the support, enthusiasm, and compassion of many extraordinary friends. Jeanine Abrons, Chia-Hung Chou, Kathy Colwell, Katherine Eade, Chris Fojtik, Gillian Glaes, Jennifer Hull, Katie Jarvis, Craig Katz and Kafryn Lieder, Rob Lewis, Camarin Porter, Bonnie Svarstad, and Salisa Westrick filled my days in Madison with joy. A warm thank-you as well to the families who welcomed me into their lives and to all of the "little friends" (two- and four-legged, furry and feathered) who made my time there memorable and who made my world a better place. How lucky I am to have found Jenni Cain, Cristy Gosney, Jean Johnson, Crystal Lykins, and Nicki Schuller so early in life and how fortunate I am that they continue to share their lives with me. Most especially, I am indebted to my sweet muse Poppie, who taught me never to overlook or fail to appreciate the beauty that is always there in front of me.

As always, I am indebted to my first and most dedicated teacher, my gifted uncle and courageous friend Fred Grout. I cannot imagine having tempered the tempest of academe so gracefully without the sage advice, gentle guidance, and persistent encouragement of my aunt, Jeanine Mount. My brother Jamie, sister Stacey, and nephew Colt have kept me grounded, and their support over the years has helped me more than they will ever know. Finally, my parents, Harry and Ninette Grout, have made innumerable sacrifices so that I might have a life of my own. They have never wavered in their faith in my abilities, they have unconditionally supported my choices, and they have believed in me even when I did not. It is with love, respect, and appreciation that I dedicate this book to them.

THE FORCE
of
BEAUTY

INTRODUCTION

A Worthy Pursuit?

"Every woman can be beautiful, if she desires it," declared the Comtesse de Norville in her manual *Behind the Scenes of Beauty: How a Woman Seduces.*[1] Although Norville claimed that any woman could be beautiful, her lofty preface, which included a poem celebrating "the first toilette," and her evocation of an aristocratic lineage directed her book at a decidedly highbrow audience. In its third edition by 1895, Norville's incredibly popular 215-page cloth breviary provided twelve chapters of advice advocating a practical approach to bodily care. The author promoted hygiene and cleanliness, as well as the discreet and informed use of artifice. She also taught women how to mix their own cosmetics, how to use commercially available products, how to arrange the *cabinet de toilette,* and how to cleanse their entire bodies. By cultivating their beauty, Norville explained, middle-class women could carry out their prescribed social function and fulfill their domestic role, thus ensuring the "happiness of the family, the joy of the household."[2]

Some forty years later, in a guide released just before World War II, another counselor offered a remarkably different appraisal of feminine self-care. Sylvie's concise 103-page *How I Make My Beauty* (1937) echoed Norville's contention that every woman could be attractive. For Sylvie, a businesswoman and beauty academy proprietor, "every woman" meant not only members of the established bourgeoisie but women of all social ranks.[3] Eschewing the flowery language and urbane philosophical discussions common in earlier manuals, Sylvie offered a straightforward set of guidelines intended to help women achieve their personal beauty. Sylvie maintained that through instruction and practice, rather than the trading of secrets, women could, as she did, make their own beauty. The idea that a woman "made" her beauty suggested that looking good was not only a performance for others, as it had been for Norville, but that it was also a personal process of becoming, involving not one's husband, family, or class, but the most intimate part of one's self.

Norville's and Sylvie's assessments illustrated broader shifts in attitudes toward feminine beauty under way in Third Republic France. Emphasizing beauty's social function, Norville echoed the late-nineteenth-century sentiment that woman's appearance, especially the middle-class woman's appearance, reflected the status, morality, and health of her family and class. Considering beauty an expression of woman's individual personality, rather than classifying it as an outward manifestation of her character, Sylvie suggested that beauty's role was not to serve others but to define the self. These guides also exposed the hidden work that went into making women beautiful. Depicting personal embellishment as a rigorous, multistage process and highlighting the tools and skills required to produce a desired "look," they portrayed beautification as a time-consuming female labor. Additionally, by characterizing beauty as work—as a task to be performed rather than an attribute divinely given—these authors undermined a key component of nineteenth-century gender ideology that considered corporeal beauty a natural, essential trait of the feminine.

Although Norville and Sylvie challenged social convention by exposing feminine beauty as a cultural production, they reiterated rather than dispelled the widely held assumption that women *should* be beautiful. Their insistence that the female body was always under construction, moreover, conveniently squared with perpetually shifting beauty expectations, especially those set forth in the fine arts. Early in the nineteenth century, Romantics established the beauty standard. Renouncing the aesthetics of artifice that had characterized eighteenth-century aristocratic beauty, Romantics connected a woman's physical beauty to her self and to her soul.[4] On the female body, beauty emerged in large, expressive eyes framed by long lashes, flowing dark hair that sharply contrasted a clear complexion highlighted by rosy cheeks, and a small, well-shaped mouth.[5] These features, which signaled purity, sexuality, refinement, and restraint in equal measure, combined to produce a beauty ideal that was paradoxically magnetic and mysterious, virtuous and seductive.

The Romantic image was eclipsed at midcentury by a revival of the classical Greek ideal, which appraised female beauty using objective, analytical ratios of proportion and symmetry. During the Third Republic, beauty experts uniformly evoked corporeal proportion (a woman's measurements), facial symmetry (the relative size and shape of facial components), and harmony (the execution, through toilette and fashion, of a woman's overall "look") as the fundamental criteria upon which to evaluate female beauty. Although the measures themselves remained constant, the standards they upheld changed frequently. In the 1870s and 1880s, for instance, the ideal female body was corseted and curvy while the face was pale, natural (devoid of cosmetics), and fresh.[6] From the 1890s until the Great War, corseted figures persisted (6 million corsets were sold in 1900), but the hourglass figure was giving way to a more streamlined, athletic build.[7] At this time, women subjected their bodies to new disciplinary regimes—more frequent and vigorous bathing, gymnastics, weight-loss regimens—and the "health" and "youth" of the slender, girlish form rivaled and eventually supplanted the "charm" and "sex appeal" of the more mature, curvaceous one.[8] In the postwar decade, the trim, youthful body triumphed as fashions dictated a flattening of form and insinuated a masculinized aesthetic via cropped hair and unisex clothing. Even as women adorned their bodies with less ornate, more comfortable clothing, however, they increasingly expressed their individual personalities more overtly through the audacious use of visible makeup. By the 1930s, then, the pale, shapely innocent of the nineteenth century had been replaced by the tanned, sleek vixen. Painted seemingly from head to toe—this was, after all, the first decade of vogue for both nail polishes and bronzers—the beauty ideal of the 1930s exuded sex appeal, exoticism, and glamour.

But how and why did feminine beauty standards evolve so dramatically during the Third Republic? To address this question, *The Force of Beauty* considers how beauty—specifically as it was achieved with the tools and strategies supplied by commercial beauty culture—posed overlapping contradictions for French women, contradictions that enabled women to simultaneously reinforce and challenge established gender norms. Nineteenth-century gender ideology dictated that women, particularly middle-class women, create themselves as visually appealing decorative objects. Moreover, because it presupposed that women were naturally inclined toward personal adornment and frivolity and because women were always on view, this ideology presumed that women embellished their bodies to satisfy the demands of others. But to what extent did women engage in beauty work to please others and to what extent did they do so for themselves? What were the social and political values attached to feminine self-care? How did those values change over the course of the Third Republic? And, how did they influence popular perceptions of feminine beauty? Moreover, how do we account for those women who derived personal pleasure from cultivating the corporeal self? Did they pose a direct threat to conventional notions of womanhood, or did they reinforce expectations regarding feminine indulgence and duty that lay at the heart of nineteenth-century gender ideology?

The Force of Beauty examines these questions by exploring how beauty both limited and liberated women. Requiring time, money, energy, and effort, beauty work undeniably extended woman's long list of daily duties. Certainly, women who could not measure up to prevailing beauty standards—for economic, aesthetic, or other reasons—risked being viewed as inferior. Meanwhile, the homogenizing effects of following trends to achieve a fashionable "look" and participating in beauty work as a matter of social convention to some extent curtailed woman's ability to distinguish herself as an individual. But for women who could participate in this work and especially for those who delighted in it, beautification facilitated self-expression and enhanced visibility. In this way, beauty offered infinite possibilities for self-invention and encouraged women to constantly see themselves anew. Thus as both a barrier to and conduit of woman's self-production, beauty was instrumental in creating the conditions of possibility for imagining womanhood.

To this end, beauty's contradictions have located it at the center of fierce contests regarding the cultural productions of and subsequent meanings attached to "womanhood" and "femininity." Deceptive in their apparent similarity, womanhood and femininity, as I employ them, delimit two related but independent explanatory concepts. Broadly conceived, womanhood signifies the embodied experiences of being a woman. Inherent in this definition is consideration of the material conditions, social institutions, discursive situations, and political positions that have framed women's lived experiences as well as an understanding of how women, through individual and collective efforts, have navigated these structures. If womanhood connotes the social in this book, femininity designates the cultural. Femininity supplies the representational language and symbolic repertoire through which womanhood becomes coherent—even while it exposes the limits of that coherence. Precisely because it occupies itself with the idea of "woman," because it perpetually calls into question what it means to be a "woman," femininity reveals womanhood as a performance. Beauty, then, in its distinctive capacity to articulate the rhetorical machinations as well as the quotidian practices through which these performances transpire, provides a privileged marker of intimate connections between the personal and the political. As such, beauty offers an especially useful conceptual framework for understanding the cultural discourses and social practices through which femininity and womanhood have been produced.

ARTIFICE AND ITS DISCONTENTS

Beauty is political. From the eighteenth century forward, cultural debates about feminine beauty, specifically as it was achieved through cosmetics use, advanced compelling connections between the personal and the political, connections that elucidated the interwoven politics of state, class, and gender. Moreover, changing views about beauty paralleled and coincided with shifting attitudes about womanhood. By the late eighteenth century, feminine beauty work was condoned so long as it demonstrated a woman's inner virtue and did not distract her from her familial duties. During the nineteenth century, it was promoted as a vehicle to good health and as a task that enabled women to embody social expectations. Finally, in the twentieth century, beauty work empowered women to experiment with new identities even as it signaled their potential subjugation within consumer societies.

Interwoven with the Enlightenment reimagining of the public sphere, late-eighteenth-century critiques of cosmetics originated in a condemnation of artifice and in a profound disenchantment with a regime that condoned it.[9] Opponents of court ostentation argued that its pompous pageantry signified the enfeebling decadence of despotism, and they evoked the aristocratic obsession with artifice as evidence of the duplicity of the ruling orders.[10] In this opaque culture of spectacle where display trumped substance, cosmetics conferred power and prestige. Courtiers, and even the royal family itself, often appeared in public wearing masks or covered in face paints. Although cosmetics effectively reinforced social disparities, they also facilitated masquerade, sexual play, gender bending, and a host of other deviant behaviors that compromised distinctions of sex and rank. Simultaneously enabling and concealing the sexual, social, and political maneuverings of ambitious courtiers, cosmetics became synonymous with aristocratic corruption.

Critics not only disparaged cosmetics because they disguised the true characters of duplicitous individuals but also because, worn by both men and women, they veiled differences between the sexes, exposing gender itself as a façade, an ever-changing costume that individuals casually "put on."[11] One of the century's most vociferous opponents of artifice, Jean-Jacques Rousseau, leveled some of his earliest criticisms at wealthy male cosmetics wearers (specifically the *petit maître,* the male counterpart of the coquette and probable predecessor to the nineteenth-century dandy). These men, who wore powder, rouge, and wigs, and who enjoyed the profligate pleasures of warm-water bathing, upset the natural order by appearing in public as indistinguishable from fashionable ladies.[12] By removing wigs (or at least adopting less extravagant ones) and washing off face paints, Rousseau asserted, French men could eradicate the effeminate associations of elite masculinity and remake themselves into virile, judicious, "manly" men.[13]

Rousseau chastised aristocratic men for their complicity in the moral and political disgrace of France, but he was even more critical of the women who, he believed, both participated in and facilitated that decline.[14] Rousseau maintained that women employed cosmetics to control the sexual economy and to secretly influence the politics of state. A painted face, he argued, masked a tainted soul, and women who painted did so only to indulge their vanity, to appease their need for attention, and to seduce, then ruin, men.[15] By linking feminine cosmetics use to unfettered sexual power, Rousseau depicted unnaturally embellished women as a threat to the social order.[16] To bring women back into the virtuous fold, Rousseau imagined Sophie, whose natural beauty exemplified her submissiveness. According to Rousseau, woman was "specially made for man's delight," and her role was to "be pleasing in his sight, to win his respect and love, to train him in childhood, to tend him in manhood, to counsel and console, to make his life pleasant and happy."[17] Moreover, because the art of pleasing "finds its physical basis in personal adornment," woman was to be charming, sexually chaste, and physically attractive, without the aid of artifice.[18] In other words, virtuous women were *naturally* beautiful.

The same ideas regarding natural beauty and woman's capacity to please espoused by eighteenth-century moralists like Rousseau found expression within a nineteenth-century liberal ideology of gender that defined woman's social role primarily as domestic and decorative. Premised on the idea that biological sex determined social behaviors, this ideology identified characteristics such as intellect, morality, and sentiment as fixed in the body. The emphasis on sex difference, moreover, made physical beauty, which was conceived narrowly as a woman's anatomical inheritance, an especially relevant marker of womanhood. Rendering her ornamental, passive, fragile, frivolous, and in need of protection, beauty justified woman's subordinate status within the family and society and qualified other equally arbitrary characteristics associated with her sex, including passionlessness and docility.

Throughout the nineteenth century, the management of women's bodies concerned lawmakers, reformers, moralists, and mothers across France. Women were expected to beautify to attract a desirable husband and were reminded constantly that their physical appearance represented the health of the family and the robustness of the middle class. Tasked with these duties, the respectable woman cultivated an ambiguous relationship with cosmetics. From a tender age, girls were groomed in class-prescribed beauty rituals. The stakes involved in executing a pleasing toilette, however, amplified once a young woman entered society. Desperate to defeat rivals on the marriage market, women increasingly relied upon *maquillage invisible*—creams, powders, and lotions—that could enhance corporeal attributes without being easily detected. Visible cosmetics, called *fards,* remained, of course, completely off-limits. Associated with actresses, prostitutes, and other women of ill-repute, rouges, kohls, and lip colors visually signaled a woman's immorality and advertised her sexual availability. Despite the respectable woman's growing reliance on invisible makeup, *fards* remained a legible marker of moral difference, sorting out the good girls from the bad.

Opinions toward artificial embellishment began to slowly change in the last decades of the nineteenth century amid fears of depopulation and national degeneracy. At this time, lawmakers, social reformers, and physicians anxious about public health and personal hygiene promoted feminine beauty work as a pathway to good health.[19] Emphasizing cleanliness over vanity, doctors and hygienists endorsed woman's use of cleansers, deodorizers, and other sanitizing agents. At the same time, the beauty industry began to manufacture safer, more effective, and less expensive beauty aids that enabled women to carry out the duties of hygienic beautification. The clean, attractive female body now performed a double duty: it embodied bourgeois values and symbolized the vitality of the French nation. An unanticipated result of legitimizing woman's use of hygienic beauty aids was that visible cosmetics—products intended to embellish without necessarily providing hygienic benefit—also became more socially acceptable. Aligning cosmetics use with health and hygiene, officials, reformers, and the beauty industry inadvertently connected artifice to middle-class respectability.

The new attitudes toward female embellishment that grew out of these efforts opened the way for a flourishing commercial beauty culture to take shape at the turn of the century. Offering women a seemingly endless array of products, services, and treatments, the beauty industry provided everything that women needed to make their own beauty. The images and discourses generated within this culture, especially those in advertisements, advice manuals, and women's periodicals, encouraged women to entertain fantasies of self. If, as Judith Butler has argued, "the body becomes its gender through a series of acts which are renewed, revised, and consolidated through time," then beauty work enabled women—through quotidian corporeal practices, the literal putting on and taking off of beauty aids—to reimagine themselves every day.[20]

Beauty culture further promoted woman's efforts to produce and to perform different versions of the self by generating culturally vibrant models of womanhood to which ordinary women aspired. Twentieth-century beauty icons—pageant queens, entertainers, models, and Hollywood starlets—openly embraced the transformative possibilities of cosmetics and modeled the malleability of female bodies for all women. Through public displays and mass-circulated images, moreover, these models reinforced the idea that women's bodies were made to be looked at, admired, and desired. Complicit in the commodification and spectacularization of the beautified, sexualized female body, beauty icons seemed to celebrate woman's ornamental status. Consequently, inundated with images of exceptionally attractive women, ordinary women strove to achieve similar looks but were all too often forced to confront their own physical limitations. Incapable of measuring up, even with the aid of beauty products, services, and procedures, average women could spend their entire lives chasing impossible dreams.

Indeed, it was the concern that commercial beauty culture indiscriminately perpetuated unattainable models of femininity that privileged appearance over substance that led twentieth-century critics to increasingly evoke beauty to mark divisions between the feminine and the feminist. In her manifesto *The Second Sex* (1949), Simone de Beauvoir argued that cosmetics use, which had by the 1940s become commonplace among French women of all social classes, reinforced woman's decorative function, turning her into an idol and a sex object.[21] The daily toilette, in particular, required time, money, and effort that took woman away from "worthy pursuits."[22] Moreover, Beauvoir maintained that beauty could not be considered an autonomous feminine act because woman's social duty was to "make a good showing." Although woman enjoyed "letting herself be seen," caring for her beauty remained a "kind of work that enables her to take possession of her person as she takes possession of her home through housework," and thus constituted a form of domestic drudgery. A few decades later, feminist scholars echoed Beauvoir's concerns and decried the psychological damage inflicted by depictions of idealized beauty, which they maintained represented male efforts to discipline women's bodies.[23] The beauty industry, they charged, intentionally cultivated corporeal dissatisfaction among average women and bound them to a market of seemingly limitless commodities intended to improve imperfect bodies. In these ways, feminists denounced cosmetics as symbols of woman's oppression within patriarchal, capitalist societies.[24]

Yet reading woman's engagement with commercial beauty culture simply as an index of her sociopolitical and economic subjugation ignores intimate linkages between the production of the feminine and the production of wide-ranging social, cultural, and political processes. During the Third Republic, womanhood was negotiated amid charged debates regarding women's sociopolitical status. Although women did not enjoy full rights of citizenship, legislation concerning divorce, property ownership, and access to earnings and savings accounts, alongside increased access to education and an expanding market that actively sought female consumers, encouraged women to pursue rights heretofore denied them.[25]

At the same time, the definition of respectable womanhood broadened, albeit marginally, to accommodate workingwomen, consuming women, and, to a lesser extent, independent, single women. As French women became more publicly visible—a process accelerated but not entirely instigated by the Great War—attention to physical appearance intensified for both sexes. Looking and being looked at became normative activities in public spaces, and, because they privileged appearing, these practices paradoxically heightened and obscured awareness of the individual. It was thus within a less restrictive, more permissive republic that nineteenth-century notions of gender fixity slowly gave way to twentieth-century notions of gender fluidity. Through the holographic lens of beauty, then, we begin to glimpse how tensions among personal bodies, social bodies, and the body politic laid bare the contradiction between formal and substantive rights that characterized the French woman's complicated relationship to republicanism.

Thus carefully scrutinizing beauty's authorizing contradiction—its uncanny ability to concurrently reinforce and upend established norms—reveals the possibilities opened up by and the perils involved in making beauty a worthy pursuit. This book examines how beauty prescribed a social duty for women, how it has been evoked to legitimize their subordinate status and to reduce them to their biological sex. But it also demonstrates how beauty has functioned as a subversive tool of feminine self-expression. Beauty in the service of others, carried out to uphold values of family, class, and nation, undeniably validated woman's ancillary social position. However, beauty as a method of self-production, as a disruptive force capable of denaturalizing the body and deessentializing sex difference, destabilized the very gender hierarchy that it supported. Understood in this way, women emerge not as passive victims of an officious beauty industry but as autonomous actors who used the tools of commercial beauty culture to transform their bodies and to transcend social convention.[26]

COMMERCIAL BEAUTY CULTURE

If beauty is political; then what, exactly, are the politics of beauty? This question, most productively considered through the lens of France's commercial beauty culture, illuminates how women's everyday practices shaped what Ilya Parkins calls the "broad sweeps of history."[27] During the Third Republic, cosmetics transformed from superfluous luxury items into reputable consumer goods. The French meanwhile entertained new ideas about femininity and beauty that opened a space for envisioning new models of womanhood.[28] These concurrent and intertwined developments created the conditions necessary for a thriving commercial beauty culture. Moreover, they shaped the discourses and practices through which ordinary women used that culture to make their own beauty. Thus the lens of commercial beauty culture not only reveals intimate connections between abstract aesthetics and the material world, but it also illustrates how these intersections, as they were articulated on and through the female body, positioned women variably within fluctuating cultural, symbolic, and commercial economies.

By "commercial beauty culture," I mean the constellation of businesses and media that interplayed with social practices and cultural discourses to produce competing models of womanhood. Businesses, including cosmetics firms, salons, and retailers ranging from department stores to one-price emporia, provided the necessary products and commercial infrastructure to support a competitive beauty market.[29] The media, namely periodicals and the cinema, used the products manufactured and distributed by these businesses to create popular models of female beauty. Meanwhile, ordinary women, influenced by advertisements, novels, and self-help manuals and who aspired to look like media-generated icons, engaged in daily beautification practices that connected them simultaneously to both media fantasies of femininity and to the industry that provided the tools required to bring those fantasies to life.

Through this tangled web of commerce and culture, I explore woman's evolving relationship to beauty as a critical site of identity construction. In so doing, I expand Kathy Peiss's definition of beauty culture as "a type of commerce and a system of meaning that helped women navigate the changing conditions of modern social experience," to consider not only how women assimilated the multifarious meanings attached to beauty or to understand how they participated in a particular form of commerce, but also to assess how beauty became embedded in the conditions of social existence itself.[30] In other words, I am interested in the various ways that beauty paradoxically reveals and conceals operations of power that structure social relationships.

Accessing these hidden operations, however, requires first dismantling and then reconstructing France's commercial beauty culture. Yet because it is expressed simultaneously in markets, material culture, social practices, and cultural discourses, commercial beauty culture as both an economy and a concept is difficult to pin down. Just as no single archival source documents its commercial development, no set of sources fully articulates its cultural contributions. The task before the scholar, then, is to assemble, analyze, and situate in dialogue a disparate array of historical sources. To uncover the workings of beauty businesses, I read hygiene manuals, professional and legal debates about the right to fabricate and distribute products, and print and poster advertisements alongside firm histories and trade journal articles. These sources reveal the major players within the industry, and they illuminate the social and economic conditions that gave rise to a viable commercial beauty culture. At the same time, I explore how cultural media—women's periodicals, self-care guides, novels, works of art, beauty contests, cinema, and advertisements—evoked the tools and products offered by this culture to produce new models of womanhood.

Additionally, I afford special attention to the commodity itself. Scholars have argued that consumer durables affect social and political change; that processes of commodification parallel advances in political democratization in some liberal democratic regimes; and that quotidian commodities structure lexicons through which objects, individuals, and societies communicate within, among, and about one another.[31] I am particularly interested in both the use value assigned to cosmetics and to the cultural meanings they transmit. On the one hand, cosmetics provide a window into the private experiences of daily life. A necessary component of woman's toilette, cosmetics decorate her living space as well as her body. Woman's reliance on these objects and her demand that they fit her lifestyle shape her relationship to commercial beauty culture and influence her attitudes toward corporeal beauty—her own as well as that of other women. On the other hand, cosmetics as value-laden cultural signifiers communicate, reinforce, and subvert commonly held social principles. Women mark their bodies with cosmetics, but in so doing they actively mimic, manipulate, or reject prevailing beauty standards. In both scenarios, women and cosmetics, subjects and objects, make one another, and, through this process, beauty becomes instrumental to carrying out the work of womanhood.[32] By considering cosmetics historical artifacts whose socioeconomic functions and multivalent cultural meanings change over time, I propose to take mundane consumer objects seriously as makers and markers of modern gender identities.[33]

Whereas some scholars have been unsympathetic to the beauty industry, identifying its goods and practices as impediments to female autonomy, I argue that beauty acts as a liberating as well as a limiting component of womanhood. Purchasing cosmetics, following expert advice, and engaging in certain rituals enabled women to challenge established norms and to take possession of their bodies in increasingly individuated ways. These same activities, however, also cost women time and money and threatened, as Beauvoir lamented, to take them away from more worthy pursuits. In the chapters that follow, I investigate the businesses and technologies that underwrote France's commercial beauty culture as well as the social practices and the professional, aesthetic, and popular discourses that provided a cultural context for femininity during the Third Republic. In so doing, I attempt to unravel the complicated relationship between the politics of womanhood and the politics of beauty.

THE CONTESTED MEANING OF BEAUTY

But what is gained, ultimately, by making beauty a worthy pursuit? Answering this question requires accounting for how both historical actors and historians have grappled with beauty's contested meanings. Depending upon context, beauty might connote an aesthetic, an economy, a form of work; but it might also signify a process, indicate a state of being, or express an idea. Understood as both naturally occurring and humanly fashioned, corporeal beauty is especially fraught. At the same time that it is invoked to define and glorify the eternal feminine and to lock women into fixed social and sexual roles, it also exposes the mutability of female bodies.

In the late nineteenth century, as part I of this book demonstrates, beauty enabled middle-class women to fulfill their social duties and to embody cultural expectations of respectability even while it undermined those duties and expectations by encouraging women to embrace their sexuality. Tasked with ensuring the health and hygiene of their reproductive bodies as well as those of their family members, middle-class women cultivated corporeal beauty to meet "new standards of cleanliness" imposed by healthcare professionals.[34] Decorative and functional, the sanitized, beautified female body now represented the social vitality of the French middle class. But even as beauty work became aligned with female respectability in this way, it continued to signal woman's sexual desire. Suggestive depictions of alluring women as nymphs, courtesans, and seductresses in the high arts blatantly exploited connections between cosmetics use and female sexuality, while more mundane discussions of beauty work found in women's periodicals and self-care manuals taught even respectable women how to transform their bodies into objects of desire.

Despite concerted efforts to reconcile respectability and female sexuality, part 2 traces how this tension became beauty's most visible, most salient contradiction in the early twentieth century. In their cultural productions—novels, essays, memoirs, public performances on stage and in print—as well as in their daily lives, exceptional women like the celebrated author and eventual beauty entrepreneur Sidonie-Gabrielle Colette seized upon this contradiction to enact new female roles. Colette explored the ways that beauty expectations placed upon women rendered them superfluous decorative objects. But in her celebration of cosmetics—their use, their utility, and their symbolic power—she also divulged how beauty facilitated and enhanced the work of becoming a woman.

Finally, as part III shows, opportunities for creative self-fashioning abounded for ordinary women in the two decades following the Great War. At this time, beauty industries across the globe began intermingling, producing new cultures of beauty along the way that came to France through exciting cultural forms. Among them, beauty contests and the cinema emerged as particularly dynamic messengers. These forms, as commercial vehicles charged with demonstrating the products available within a global market and as cultural sites devoted to exhibiting the most current embodiments of feminine beauty, mediated woman's relationship to interwar commercial beauty cultures. Moreover, connecting women to transnational commodity circuits as well as to international beauty ideals, beauty contests and cinema sanctioned the unapologetic public display of female bodies while enabling French women, especially metropolitan, middle-class women, to see themselves and to "be seen" as part of a broader, global phenomenon of modern womanhood.

For historians, then, beauty as a worthy academic pursuit not only provides a compelling analytical lens through which to understand the developments above but also sheds new light on complex, often hidden operations involved in producing and performing a gendered self. Daily beauty practices—cleansing and embellishing the body with commodities, applying skin-care therapies, even traveling to the salon or the institute for corporeal maintenance treatments—functioned as constituting acts, which enabled women to create desirable self-images.[35] These practices also, significantly, revealed the centrality of the body to modern constructions of the gendered self. Functioning simultaneously as a "layer of experience, site of subjectivity, or representation of the self or social collectivity," the body, according to Kathleen Canning, offers insight into the history of everyday life and points to how quotidian experiences are gendered.[36] Moreover, because identity is not stable but, as Butler asserts, "tenuously constituted in time," a critical analysis of beauty work reveals the nuanced ways that mundane practices create identities.

The Force of Beauty thus chronicles the many ways that beauty has marked the feminine. I analyze these demarcations first by figuring beauty practices as constituting acts. I show how daily choices about personal care, though executed within frameworks over which women had limited control, were nevertheless assertions of individuality rooted in a politics of the everyday. Attentive to beauty's fraught contradictions, I also examine the myriad ways that beauty has revealed the insidious channels through which imbricated power hierarchies, particularly those of state, class, and gender, have found visual expression on and through marked female bodies. Through these explorations, I suggest that beauty not only marked the production, practice, and performance of femininity, but, by providing women with the tools and strategies to "make their beauty," it also invited them to envision womanhood in new ways.

PART I

Respectable Beauty

> Woman is quite within in her rights, indeed she is even accomplishing a kind of duty, when she devotes herself to appearing magical and supernatural; she has to astonish and charm us; as an idol, she is obliged to adorn herself and to be adored. . . . Thus, if you will understand me aright, face-painting should not be used with the vulgar, unavowable object of imitating fair Nature and of entering into competition with youth. It has moreover been remarked that artifice cannot lend charm to ugliness and can only serve beauty. . . . Maquillage has no need to hide itself or to shrink from being suspected; on the contrary, let it display itself, at least if it does so with frankness and honesty.
>
> —Charles Baudelaire, "In Praise of Cosmetics"

In his collection of essays *The Painter of Modern Life* (1863), Charles Baudelaire joyfully celebrated woman's right to employ artifice. Not only did he appreciate woman's well-executed toilette, but he regarded it as a "kind of duty" that she was "obliged" to perform. Baudelaire condemned the "errors of the field of aesthetics [that] spr[u]ng from the eighteenth-century's false premises." He argued instead that artifice should not endeavor to replicate nature or recapture youth. It should be worn "with frankness and honesty" and need only serve the wearer herself.[1] Baudelaire's essay appeared at the height of the Second Empire, when artifice experienced a new period of vogue among the elites of Louis Napoleon Bonaparte's imperial court. Nevertheless, the poet's promotion of cosmetics, and the vibrant, feminized commodity culture that they signaled, was not yet enthusiastically accepted by a status quo that considered them false prophets, monikers of a duplicitous character, and tools of deception.

During the eighteenth century, cosmetics were important commodities in France's growing luxury trades. Yet, because their use remained the prerogative of elites who possessed both the capital to purchase them and the time to use them, cosmetics operated as more than objects for purchase. They functioned as value-laden cultural signifiers that articulated the social and political hierarchies of the Ancien Régime. Within this culture of appearances, the use of artifice was carried out by social prescription and worked to reinforce rank-based proprietary norms. Elites equated whiteness with *civilisation* and *politesse*, and so to appear *propre* they painted their lips dark red and powdered their hair and wigs. The elite toilette established a social uniform that distinguished the aristocracy from the unbathed, unruly masses as well as from the uncultured middling sort. In this way, cosmetics became synonymous with aristocratic privilege, and they offered a visible template of social difference—a perceptible lexicon of power that could be easily read and decoded by even the most illiterate French men and women.

In the nineteenth century, however, a new commercial beauty culture emerged that rendered feminine beauty an essential precept of middle-class respectability. Promoting sanitary self-care as evidence of the middle-class woman's restraint, propriety, and good taste, this culture established beauty as a legitimate and necessary form of woman's work. Whereas her self-centered elite predecessors overindulged the female body, languishing in warm-water baths, covering every inch of skin with perfumes and paints, the practical middle-class woman conscientiously maintained her body by carrying out a sensible, hygienic toilette. Despite efforts to sanitize artifice, however, the specter of the decadent aristocrat continued to haunt beauty practices and discourses: advertisements featured cultural elites (actresses, socialites); lavish product packages connoted luxury; and advisors and counselors often claimed noble ancestry. But if the target consumer was bourgeois, why so blatantly connect beauty to its aristocratic origins? Whereas practical goods secured markets based solely on utility, luxury items, according to Stephen Gundle, "relied heavily on the ideas that were associated with them, in particular the promise of magical transformation or instant escape from the constraints of everyday life."[2] Boasting a seemingly infinite array of magical products and transformative practices, France's commercial beauty culture certainly encouraged middle-class women to entertain "supernatural" fantasies.

Part I examines how the commercial beauty culture that emerged in nineteenth-century France constructed beauty as both a necessary female duty and an indulgent feminine pleasure. The first chapter investigates how beauty businesses (cosmetics firms, hair salons, institutes, product fabricators, and distributors) worked alongside health-care professionals (doctors, hygienists) to make beauty work socially acceptable. Growth in the beauty trade was fueled by developments within the chemical and pharmaceutical industries, the revolution in retailing, and advancements in the field of advertising. Significantly, these transformations transpired within a France increasingly anxious about national hygiene and public health. In the crusade against disease and depopulation, doctors and hygienists authored numerous self-care manuals. These manuals legitimized woman's use of artifice by aligning it with good health and personal hygiene. This endorsement, along with the influx of safer, less toxic, more affordable products into the market, equipped women with the tools and the rationale for ministering to their bodies. Promoting beauty work as an enjoyable and necessary female labor, health-care professionals aligned corporeal care with middle-class respectability and fostered new attitudes about the female body.

Beauty did not only require work; it also performed important cultural work. Chapter 2 explores how the work of beauty exposed critical tensions between the discursive production of femininity and embodied practices of womanhood. Nineteenth-century gender ideology produced the feminine through exclusionary discourses that located woman's social identity in her sexed body. Attributing appearance, character, and intellect exclusively to woman's biology, these discourses used sex to naturalize gender differences and to establish woman's place in the social order. By the late nineteenth century, the Nineteenth-Century Venus, the Grand Coquette, and the Beauty Countess revealed that femininity, like beauty, was not a biological inheritance but a carefully choreographed social performance. Importantly, these models posed alternatives to middle-class womanhood at the same time that they expanded the boundaries of respectability. The cosmetically enhanced, publicly nude Venus, whose sexual availability signaled a social threat, also illustrated how women could create themselves as both objects and subjects of desire. The glamorous Grand Coquette, embodied by the actress/celebrity and ridiculed for her sexual promiscuity, was also admired for her extravagant beauty. Finally, the humble Beauty Countess, who posed as the pampered aristocrat, cultivated desire and encouraged indulgence by couching beauty in the middle-class language of industry.

Ultimately, beauty work and the work of beauty reconfigured the relationship between womanhood and respectability. Beauty experts connected self-care to scientific progress, personal hygiene, and public health. They reiterated the belief that women were made to please, to be decorative objects and familial trophies. And they proposed to reinscribe the female body into the service of class and nation. Yet in its tools and function, commercial beauty culture undermined the notion that beauty was natural, somehow rooted in woman's biology. Rather than portray beauty as an essential state of being, self-care manuals, breviaries, advice columns, and other cultural discourses exposed the diligent effort required to make women beautiful. Commercial beauty culture, like Baudelaire, tasked women with the "duty" of beautification; however, it also provided the tools necessary—hygiene and embellishment aids, instruction manuals, models to emulate, and commercial sites—to perform these labors. By 1900, French women were not only expected to "astonish and charm" but also to cleanse and to sanitize. In its own praise of cosmetics, France's commercial beauty culture made the pursuit of beauty respectable at the fin de siècle.

1

Beauty Work

Is it a crime to want to always please and to be loved?
And to achieve this using the most graceful tricks?
—Vicomtesse de Réville, *La Parisienne en 1900*

In the fifteenth edition of his popular health and hygiene manual *La beauté chez l'homme et chez la femme* (1891), Dr. Paul Marrin explained to his predominantly middle-class readers that using artifice to embellish the body was a "question of aesthetics and public hygiene."[1] For much of the nineteenth century, middle-class men and women associated artifice (especially artificial agents used to enhance the body) with moral corruption and sexual promiscuity. After all, it was only the dandy, the prostitute, the actor, or the imperial ingénue who dared wear grease paints and heavy powders in public. At first glance, then, Marrin's manual appeared to challenge prevailing attitudes toward cosmetics' use. Yet, by the late nineteenth century, numerous health-care professionals endorsed the middle-class woman's use of commercial beauty aids, and, like Marrin, they linked public hygiene with personal aesthetics.

By the fin de siècle, health-care professionals, primarily physicians and hygienists, made beauty work respectable by envisioning it as middle-class woman's work. Amid national initiatives aimed at curtailing the spread of disease and replenishing an aging populace, health-care professionals proposed practices that connected individual, particularly feminine, cleanliness with the collective welfare. Attributing stagnant population growth not only to disease but also to the growing accessibility of contraceptives and even to the indifference of French mothers, health-care professionals published self-care manuals that sought to cleanse and regulate the reproductive female body.[2] Article I of the law of February 19, 1902, for example, demonstrated state efforts to monitor public health through the regulation of private spaces. The law explicitly targeted "maladies transmissibles" (communicable diseases), addressed problems related to public sanitation, and sought to ensure the "cleanliness of houses and their residents." Advocating salubrious practices, authorizing the use of commercial beauty aids, and targeting women as arbiters of familial hygiene, these manuals legitimized the middle-class woman's beauty regimen by placing her body in the service of family and nation.

To no small degree, the fabrication and commercialization of new health and beauty products proved important by-products of and corollaries to national public health initiatives. The booming beauty industry that emerged in France at this time offered middle-class women a plethora of new products that promised to cleanse, sanitize, and beautify. On the advice of health-care professionals, women increasingly relied upon commercial cleansers, soaps, and deodorants to protect themselves and their families from germs. They employed professionally fabricated tonics, pastes, and elixirs to cleanse the skin, hair, and teeth. And, eager to enhance their physical appearance, women applied powders, creams, and serums to their clean bodies.

As concerns about public health escalated at the fin de siècle, health-care experts and beauty industry insiders increasingly equated beauty work with middle-class respectability. Doctors and hygienists authored countless self-care manuals. These manuals, which grew in number from twelve produced between 1800 and 1875 to seventy published between 1875 and 1900 (in the United States, England, and France collectively), echoed the call for clean, reproductive female bodies.[3] Moreover, they discursively linked feminine beauty with personal, familial, and national health to promote corporeal care as a socially acceptable, even necessary, form of middle-class woman's work. At the same time, by correlating beauty with hygiene, these manuals legitimized the respectable woman's use of artifice and encouraged her to envision herself as a desirous and desiring individual. While health-care professionals sanctioned the middle-class woman's pursuit of health and beauty, France's commercial beauty culture provided her with the tools to achieve it. Fabricators manufactured safer, less toxic aids; department stores, beauty institutes, and hair salons provided new retail outlets that made products easily accessible; and image advertisements portrayed beautification as both a glamorous indulgence and a necessary chore. Thus, under the guidance of health-care professionals and in conjunction with France's burgeoning commercial beauty culture, beauty became essential to the work of respectable middle-class womanhood.

BEAUTY IN THE SERVICE OF FAMILY AND NATION

French health-care professionals long promoted hygienic bodily care. Amid mounting concerns about population decline and growing anxieties about the health of French families, their efforts intensified. By the end of the nineteenth century, the healthy body became the focus of two major public health initiatives: the campaign to combat the spread of communicable diseases—specifically tuberculosis and syphilis; and the effort to repopulate the nation following crushing military defeat in the Franco-Prussian War (1870). While physician-legislators labored to improve public works, living conditions, and urban sanitation, other health-care professionals concentrated their efforts on the care of individual, particularly female, bodies. National debates about depopulation and disease frequently devolved into impassioned arguments about female fertility and maternal responsibility. As woman's relationship to the state was becoming understood largely in terms of maternity, her value to the nation came to reside in her clean, moral, reproductive body. Echoing this sentiment, health-care professionals authored dozens of personal-care manuals that sought to discipline the middle-class woman's body. By "extending diagnosis from the bodily to the social organism," health-care professionals placed the middle-class woman's body firmly in the service of the family and the nation.[4]

Indeed, health-care professionals were particularly well positioned to disseminate such messages. Medicine's professional prestige rose after 1870 because of falling mortality rates in hospitals, the enhanced reputation of medical schools in Paris, and doctors' better understanding of disease. At the same time, health-care professionals themselves came to exercise greater influence in French politics. Between 1870 and 1914, 358 physicians and 36 pharmacists won election as deputies or senators.[5] Since the revolution of 1789, French physicians played a more influential role in politics than their European counterparts, but that role greatly expanded under the Third Republic, when many doctors welcomed political activism as a way to enhance the prestige and authority of their profession.[6] Thus, health-care professionals derived professional legitimacy from their access to medical knowledge as well as from their relationship to the state. Even as physicians won the esteem of voters in the political realm, however, they still had to convince ordinary citizens of the value of their medical advice. One way that they did this was by authoring manuals that enabled them, by dispelling popular myths and demonstrating the personal and social benefits of self-care, to exercise disciplinary power over the docile bodies of individual men and women.[7]

In these manuals, health-care professionals associated feminine morality with sexual hygiene. Despite strides in identifying and treating syphilis, between 1890 and 1914, an estimated 13–15 percent of all Parisian males presented symptoms of the disease and 1 million individuals nationwide were believed to be infected.[8] By 1900, scientists had definitively connected the transmission of syphilis to sexual practices, specifically to illicit and venal sex.[9] Armed with this information, hygienists denounced nonprocreative sex as perverse, blamed the female prostitute for polluting the population, and linked disease to the larger problem of population decline. Syphilis and tuberculosis affected all European populations; however, these diseases were particularly troubling to the French because they fueled anxieties about national degeneration.[10] Between 1850 and 1910, the French population increased by only 3.4 million, from 35.7 million to 39.1 million.[11] Notwithstanding this increase, French parents failed to produce as many babies as couples in other parts of Europe, notably Germany and Britain. Furthermore, the French population was aging. Individuals under the age of twenty-one accounted for only 34.9 percent of the population, compared with 43.7 percent in Germany.[12] To make matters worse, nationwide deaths outnumbered births by three hundred in each year between 1891 and 1895.[13] In light of these developments, physician legislators and social hygienists urged middle-class women to produce healthy babies and to inculcate their children with the values of cleanliness.

For most of the nineteenth century, however, popular concerns related to the spread of disease prevented French men and women from fully submerging their bodies in water.[14] Even as late as the fin de siècle, partial baths that enabled local washing (and that could be easily assembled for use) were preferred over full-body baths. Resistance to full-body bathing was further evidenced in quotidian hair-care practices. Until the widespread acceptance of shampooing, hair care involved, for men, the periodic application of pomades; and for women, untangling, brushing, and braiding prior to bedtime. On occasion for both sexes, it warranted cleansing powders or soapy sponges applied over the head. Frequent shampooing became a viable cleansing option only with the proliferation of easy-to-use hair-care lotions in the early twentieth century.[15]

Despite their vehement advocacy of head-to-toe corporeal cleansing, health-care professionals themselves had only recently learned of the benefits of full-body submersion.[16] The introduction of Pasteurian science in the 1870s and the development of microbiology in the 1880s revealed water as a first line of defense against germs. Germ theory enabled scientists to bring cholera, smallpox, and typhoid under control, and it imparted a new understanding of disease transmission. Convinced that it prevented rather than spread disease, health-care professionals presented full-body washing as the cornerstone of cleanliness. "General cleanliness of the body," Dr. Ris-Paquot explained, "requires that from time to time we take a full bath. This is not an act of vanity, but a precept of hygiene, aimed at cleansing the skin."[17] Limited access to indoor plumbing meant that the average French person bathed two to three times per year. Dr. Ernest Monin, however, suggested that bathing should occur "every week" or at least "every fifteen days." He added that the temperature of the bath should range between 28 and 32 degrees centigrade to achieve optimal cleanliness. He also described a variety of infusions (oils, herbs, sea salts) that might enhance the bathing experience.[18] Promoting cleanliness as a virtue rather than a vanity, Monin and Ris-Paquot portrayed regular bathing as the foundation of good health.

Health-care professionals also envisioned beauty work as a fundamental component of middle-class womanhood. It was, as Dr. Monin explained, "the eternal mission of woman to please man . . . by acquiring and augmenting her beauty."[19] Authors began from the basic assumption that women needed (even desired) instruction in the daily care of their bodies. Once they established this imperative, writers then addressed particular cleansing techniques and product usage. Manuals varied widely in length and focus, but they commonly fit into one of three categories: the comprehensive dictionary, the practical guide, or the intimate conversation. Written in the third person and assuming an objective tone, dictionaries or encyclopedias exposed readers to a variety of personal-care regimens. Practical guides also informed readers about available products and valuable techniques. Characterized by step-by-step advice on how to carry out hygienic regimes and on how to mix and apply beauty aids, practical guides proved more instructive than dictionaries. Although they tackled similar issues, intimate guides did not dictate advice but explicitly engaged the reader so as to bring her into the expert's confidence. All three manual types characterized feminine beauty work not as a vain frivolity but as a serious, socially significant enterprise.

In their pursuit of cleanliness, women could rely on hygiene dictionaries. In 1826, César Gardeton published his *Dictionnaire de la beauté: La toilette sans danger.* Gardeton's guide offered readers "easy precepts" for "maintaining good health" and for "prolonging one's existence in an agreeable manner."[20] This extensive *dictionnaire* devoted six pages to different types of baths, forty-four pages to *eau* in various forms, several pages to *pommades* and *poudres,* and it provided a twenty-page exposition on corporeal beauty. Gardeton did not include a formulary of ingredients that could be mixed into beauty aids, but he did indicate several Parisian establishments where readers could purchase such products. For example, one could find a good *crème de cathay* at a little shop on the rue Saint-Honoré or a reliable *pommade des francs* at the perfumer located on the rue Saint-Martin.

Readers who wanted more than mere descriptions could turn to detailed practical manuals for additional advice. In *Hygiène, médicine, parfumerie, pharmacie* (1894), Dr. Ris-Paquot offered a "book of remedies used by doctors and pharmacists." Drawing on "scientific expertise," he instructed readers on personal care at all four stages of life: childhood, adolescence, adulthood, and old age. Like Gardeton, Ris-Paquot advised on bathing technique and included scores of recipes for hair cleansers, tooth elixirs, and cosmetics.[21] Perhaps the most prolific manual author, Dr. Monin published no fewer than two hundred manuals (some of these were undoubtedly reissues) between 1875 and 1930. Monin covered a variety of topics from the treatment of skin maladies to curing stomach upset and compounding simple medicines. Moreover, his manuals were frequently revised, with new editions reaching the market within just a few years after their original publication. Monin's manuals generally included five to twenty chapters and discussed a range of diverse topics: dry vs. oily skin, the art of shampooing, dental care, and feminine hygiene. His best-selling *L'hygiène de la beauté: Formulaire cosmétique* (1896) spanned sixteen chapters and consisted of 360 pages. Individual chapters addressed skin hygiene, the care of the mouth and teeth, and the fabrication of perfumes and cosmetics. Within these chapters, Monin provided step-by-step instructions for how to carry out one's daily ablutions. In the chapter devoted to facial cleansing, for instance, he extolled the benefits of glycerin and lanoline while warning against soaps that dried the skin. Likewise, in his section on cosmetics, he counseled against the "abuse of alkaline products," which, if used inappropriately, could have horrible effects on the user's appearance.[22]

Monin's manuals not only introduced readers to valuable hygienic practices; they also counseled readers on the fabrication of homemade health and beauty aids. Women had long concocted their own creams and serums in their home kitchens. Rather than discourage them from continuing to do so, Monin offered a compromise: he urged them to seek the advice of pharmacists and chemists when attempting to make their own cleansers and creams. He also provided extensive, meticulous instructions on how to mix and use homemade agents. In *Hygiène de la femme,* Monin included at least fifty recipes for creams, serums, and pomades; while in *L'hygiène de la beauté,* he provided a 137-page cosmetic formulary.[23]

An extension of the practical manual, the intimate guide was an option for women who desired a more personal connection with the health-care expert. The Doctoresse M. Schultz structured her *Hygiène générale de la femme,* published in 1903, as a series of questions and answers between herself and her reader. Asking, for example, "What is the hygiene of the skin?," she identified three elements: "1. Cleanliness is the main point of skin hygiene; 2. Fashion clothing comes next; finally, 3. Caring for exposed areas, the face, hands, and hair." Schultz not only adopted a personal tone in her manual; she also unequivocally associated woman's bodily hygiene with her moral character. She argued that the "moral equilibrium of the individual reflects on her physical health." Moreover, women who cared for their bodies were more attractive to potential partners because they looked "fresh," "happy," "moral," and "pleasing."[24] Once a woman married and bore children, it became her wifely and maternal duty to tutor her husband and offspring in proper personal hygiene practices. Schultz made this obligation explicit by addressing her manual expressly "to women, educators of children and young girls."[25] Tending to her body and teaching her family hygienic practices, a mother could help combat disease and depopulation—serving the interests of both her family and the state in the process. Connecting the physical with the moral, health-care professionals like Schultz legitimized the respectable woman's attention to her body.

Despite lingering middle-class associations between artifice and moral corruption, health-care professionals also began to endorse woman's use of cosmetics. Since the eighteenth century, doctors numbered among the most vocal opponents of cosmetics.[26] They were attuned to concerns that cosmetics use led to sexual promiscuity, and they railed against "charlatans" and "magicians" who peddled dangerous compounds to unsuspecting clients.

They also criticized the injurious application procedures practiced by wearers themselves. Doctors agreed with critics who maintained that cosmetics disfigured the feminine visage, and they took issue with the clogging properties of greases and paints. By the late nineteenth century, however, they promoted the use of nontoxic, commercially fabricated cosmetics as a steppingstone not to moral degradation but to good health.

Playing on the widely held belief that the middle-class woman's social role was to please her family and to represent her class, health-care professionals gradually divested cosmetics of their negative connotation. Early in the nineteenth century, P. J. Saint Ursin and A. Caron taught middle-class women how to use cosmetic products discreetly. In *L'ami des femmes* (1804), Saint Ursin advocated cosmetics use as long as women employed them in pursuit of personal good health and familial happiness. A. Caron's guide *Toilette des dames ou encyclopédie de la beauté* (1806) advised that women could and should use cosmetics because the social harmony of the sexes depended upon feminine beauty. Caron argued that, because the female's appearance reflected the respectability as well as the class status of her family, she must strive to be at all times beautiful and clean.

Monin's guides further developed the connection among cleanliness, artifice, and respectability by teaching women how to select commercially manufactured health and beauty aids. He counseled women to purchase products that replaced harmful mineral components with animal and vegetable derivatives. When women were choosing a *poudre de riz* (one of the most commonly used cosmetics of the time), Monin recommended that they opt for products composed of "chalk compound, talc, bismuth, alabaster, zinc oxide, or magnesium carbonate." He considered these ingredients "generally inoffensive" because they were "rarely mixed with toxic substances" that could damage the skin and eyes. He devised classification systems that helped users determine product toxicity and included instructions for the appropriate application. Monin suggested that women use cosmetics with "prudence and caution," and he urged them to apply high-quality products in ways that emphasized "the freshness of traits" while suppressing signs of "dullness and fatigue." He then went on to warn against the "habitual use of fards" (paints, kohls, and stains), which he regarded as "contrary to hygiene" because it could impede pore respiration, damage the skin, and make women look like caricatures from the theater.[27]

Obsessed with creating the *appearance* of natural beauty, health-care professionals encouraged women to use *maquillage invisible.* Products such as powders, creams, and lotions that embellished without detection were touted in manuals for providing a "natural look." These products, moreover, offered an important counter to *fards* that masked a woman's face. *Maquillage invisible* enabled respectable women to enhance rather than hide what nature gave them. By condoning its usage, health-care professionals acknowledged the middle-class woman's interest in beautification (after all, woman's concern about personal adornment was generally accepted as part of the female nature). Yet they were careful to sanction *maquillage invisible* only when it did not conflict with middle-class values. In short, a woman could experiment with cosmetics so long as she did so to serve a hygienic, moral, or social function.

In *La beauté chez l'homme et chez la femme,* Dr. Marrin moved beyond *maquillage invisible* to endorse the judicious use of visible cosmetics. Like many of his colleagues, Marrin encouraged the scientific consumption of artificial products. His lengthy full-body makeover guide (complete with highbrow aesthetic commentary, practical advice, and safe, hygienic recipes for a variety of cosmetics) concerned itself not with whether artifice was socially permissible, but whether users understood product toxicity and quality. Marrin's concern was reflected in his broad definition of cosmetics as "all of the preparations destined to conserve the freshness and the beauty of those parts of the body that are visible." Like Monin, Ris-Paquot, and Schultz, Marrin favored using a "light, supple, and nonirritating" *poudre de riz* that "adds to the skin" in lieu of paints and kohls that covered over it. Although he cautioned against the harmful ingredients found in many brightly colored *fards,* he did not proscribe their use, but rather recommended mixing them with less toxic agents.

Marrin made these concessions in part because he understood the allure of color. He was sympathetic to "certain women who abuse makeup" insofar as he recognized them as women who "desire[d] to please." But he also realized that just as cosmetics once distinguished aristocrats from their social inferiors, they now provided a legible, visible marker of distinction between certain types of women. Cosmetics, if used discreetly, could subtly suggest sexual attractiveness by masking imperfections and highlighting natural attributes; however, if used to excess, they could just as easily advertise sexual promiscuity. He expressly warned that "a face painted excessively always inspires repulsion rather than admiration," and he assured his readers that "the face gains a certain charm when discreetly embellished." In his appraisal, cosmetically enhanced feminine beauty should be neither crass nor ostentatious but subtle and admirable.[28]

Conceptualizing the female body as a privileged site for rehabilitating the nation, health-care professionals united hygiene and beauty with civic responsibility. Manuals taught middle-class women how to sanitize and discipline their bodies, encouraged them to produce healthy children, and instructed them on how to implement salubrious practices within the family. Moreover, if used appropriately, products devoted to cleansing and beautification would help mothers carry out these feminine responsibilities. Health-care professionals attempted to regulate the use of toxic mixing agents and to educate readers about the health dangers that harmful beauty aids posed. They provided women with safe alternatives to commonly used ingredients, and they implored them to seek out pharmacists, chemists, and other medical professionals for reliable mixing advice. At the same time, however, they endorsed the middle-class woman's use of cosmetics. In a twist of irony, it was through authorizing woman's use of *maquillage invisible* that health-care professionals inadvertently facilitated the social acceptance of visible cosmetics. Thus, by linking hygiene with beauty, health-care professionals helped legitimize the middle-class woman's reliance on artifice while conferring a degree of respectability onto previously suspect products and practices.

THE BUSINESS OF BEAUTY

If health-care professionals made the pursuit of personal care respectable, then beauty businesses made it safe, easy, and pleasurable. Throughout the nineteenth century, consumer demand for commercially manufactured health and beauty products increased steadily. However, within the context of the health and hygiene campaigns of the late nineteenth century, perfumery sales surged dramatically. In 1836, perfumers reported annual sales at 12 million francs; 26 million in 1866; and, by 1900, French consumers spent 90 million francs each year on perfumery products.[29] Perfumery sales increased 120 percent between 1836 and 1866 and another 250 percent between 1866 and 1900.[30]

In addition to growing consumer demand, developments in the manufacture, regulation, and distribution of personal-care aids transformed the

French beauty industry into a competitive commercial enterprise. Fabricators benefitted tremendously from advancements in the field of chemistry. They learned how to readily identify harmful agents, how to manipulate natural ingredients, and how to create synthetic compounds that made finished products safer and more stable. At the same time, state-recognized professional organizations sought to regulate the production and distribution of these items. Regulation ensured product quality and enabled perfumers, coiffeurs, and even fashion designers to join chemists and pharmacists in the fabrication of personal-care products. While perfumers expanded their offerings beyond *eau de toilettes,* colognes, and musk to include scented powders, colorful *fards,* and body oils, coiffeurs carved out a market niche by mixing their own hair tonics, cleansers, and dyes. Following the example of the English designer George Worth, fashion houses increasingly introduced beauty aids as part of their seasonal collections. Moreover, as professional battles ensued over the right to manufacture personal-care aids, new retail outlets emerged. Consumers who traditionally purchased products from the neighborhood apothecary or mixed them personally in a homemade kitchen laboratory could now buy the latest, most fashionable aids at the department store, the beauty institute, or the hair salon. Changes in the manufacture, regulation, and distribution of personal-care items revolutionized the beauty business while confirming that beauty work was the business of middle-class women.

Given the scant regulation of the fabrication of health and beauty aids in the nineteenth century, many cosmetics were compounded using toxic, sometimes deadly, ingredients.[31] Rouge, for example, was composed of everything from cinnabar (red mercury reduced to a powder/sulfur) to red lead or alkali metals like alum. And, even when made from vegetable agents like catharme or sandalwood, beauty aids were often distilled with alcohol, vinegar, or goose grease. These practices began to change when fabricators discovered how to manufacture safer products. For example, the chemist Marcellin Berthelot's synthesis of organic bodies enabled the Belgian scientist Ernst Solvay to modify soap making. Solvay's innovation involved employing the by-products of chemical reactions produced when sodium hydroxide was extracted from water and salt. In 1862, Solvay patented this procedure and began to inexpensively manufacture and sell his hygienically effective "Solvay" soap. Fabricators also replaced natural agents (goose grease, food additives) with more stable synthetic ones (zinc oxide, petroleum). This switch enabled them to rationalize product formulae and to achieve the consistency necessary to inexpensively mass-produce the primary ingredients used in most products.[32] Developments in compounding and fabrication within these burgeoning industries not only made products safer but also increased the quantity and types of aids available to consumers.

Chemists were not alone in the manufacture of safer cosmetics. Apothecaries, who had long been engaged in the fabrication and distribution of health and beauty aids, accompanied them in this endeavor. Indeed, before 1850, pharmacists enjoyed almost complete control over the commercial beauty market. A new image of the pharmacist as a scientifically oriented professional emerged in 1777 with the creation of the Collège de pharmacie. Founded in Paris, the college united apothecaries into a powerful corporate body. Moreover, Article XXV of the law of 21 germinal an XI (April 11, 1803) established the practitioner's rights and obligations and gave state-licensed pharmacists a monopoly over the preparation and sale of *médicaments* (medications).[33] The law defined *médicaments* explicitly as preparations that were listed in the official Codex, prescribed by doctors, or recognized and approved by the Medical Academy. The intent of the law was to rid France of the numerous "secret remedy" drugs in circulation and to provide a professionally managed drug formulary. In their *officines,* pharmacists compounded and dispensed hygiene and beauty aids alongside medicines, cleansers, and even pet food. They also counseled clients in the selection of safe agents and often demonstrated appropriate mixing techniques. Thus it was as mediators between clients and compounds that pharmacists established their professional place within France's diversifying beauty market.

Hairdressers soon joined pharmacists in these activities. Coiffeurs found newly available chemical agents easier to acquire and manipulate, and, once they secured long-lasting, synthetic ingredients, they began implementing new techniques that enabled them to create less toxic hair tonics, lotions, and pomades. They even began experimenting with new agents themselves so that they could offer a wider range of services and products to their clients. Hairdressing evolved from a family enterprise in which stylists devoted themselves to haircutting and wig making for a small number of bourgeois and aristocratic patrons into an organized profession hallmarked by the establishment of la Chambre des coiffeurs de Paris in 1873. Once professionalized, hairdressers opened schools and salons throughout France, and they began writing about their craft, publishing some sixty journals between 1890 and 1950. They challenged pharmacy's *médicament* monopoly by mixing and selling a wide range of health and beauty aids (shampoo sec, toothpaste, and soap) to customers of their own.[34]

In the years leading up to the Great War, hairdressers became so successful in their efforts that they found themselves involved in legal disputes with incensed pharmacists. Both groups argued that the products they sold defined their professional identity. Coiffeurs claimed that they had the right to mix products because they were experts trained in the art of caring for hair. Pharmacists, conversely, sought to retain their exclusive rights to the fabrication and distribution of all *médicaments* as promised by the law of April 1803. On July 20, 1909, a Lille pharmacist took the coiffeur Arthur Lefebvre to court for the illegal sale of pilocarpine, a substance classified as a *médicament*. The prosecutor argued that by selling the product, Lefebvre had illegally practiced pharmacy and encroached upon the rights of state-licensed pharmacists. Lefebvre was ultimately acquitted, but his case was important because it illustrated how disputes over the right to manufacture beauty products marked professional boundaries within the beauty industry.[35] That the state also became involved in these quarrels demonstrated how competitive and lucrative the trade in beauty had become by the early twentieth century.

Indeed, debates continued outside of the courtroom as spokesmen for both hairdressers and pharmacists aired their grievances in professional journals. After Lefebvre's trial, the publicist Jacques Dhur submitted an editorial to the trade journal *La parfumerie moderne* in January 1910. In it he asked, "What crime has the hairdresser committed? . . . [H]e has simply sold a fabulous lotion intended to protect hair."[36] Further, he alleged, the existing law was "ridiculous" and "outdated." It made, he claimed, "simple good sense" that a coiffeur, who earned his living selling hair and beauty products and who spent "all of his time occupied with hair," should not need to rely on a pharmacist to fabricate products that he was capable of making himself.

Despite Dhur's assurances, pharmacists had real cause for concern: many products that coiffeurs used contained toxic, even lethal ingredients. Shampooing sec, for example, a dry cleanser that left the hair soft to the touch, was composed primarily of kerosene—this concoction was not only flammable but filled salons (and, when dumped down drains, sewer systems) with toxic fumes. It was with these concerns in mind that André Langrand, the président du Syndicat général des pharmaciens de France, responded to Dhur in *La perfumerie moderne*. In favor of improving existing legislation, Langrand would not, however, "support a law that permits hairdressers to handle poisonous compounds of which they know neither the effects nor the dangers. The free sale of medicaments was tolerated in France at one time, but that was before chemistry gave us the innumerable poisons that we have today." Allowing hairdressers to handle certain medicaments, he continued, "would be disastrous. . . . Although the current law is flawed . . . and might necessitate an overhaul, some judicious amendments have proven vital and must remain."[37] In his rebuttal, Langrand expressed concern for the safety of both hairdressers and their clients. Pharmacists should retain the right to mix and distribute *médicaments* not merely because they were legally entitled to economically profit from that business but also because they were trained professionals who worked in the public interest. Despite these objections, hairdressers were not prohibited from creating their own products. They would prove formidable competitors in the expanding beauty market.

The novice chemist-turned–hair expert Eugene Schueller would rank among the most important beauty professionals to emerge in the early twentieth century. Born in Alsace-Lorraine on March 20, 1881, Schueller was a student living in Paris by 1900. Schueller became involved in the business of hair care when he accepted a challenge from a Parisian hairdresser. The coiffeur asked Schueller's college chemistry class to create a product that would make hair more manageable. The inexperienced but enthusiastic student began experimenting in his home kitchen, laboring night after night until he created "L'Auréole," a *teinture capillaire* that proved to be the first nonabrasive, semipermanent hair dye. The success of L'Auréole among Parisian coiffeurs encouraged Schueller to continue mixing hair tonics and serums. In 1909, the young chemist registered his brand with the Société française des teintures inoffensives pour cheveux under the new company name, L'Oréal.[38]

L'Oréal revolutionized the manufacture and distribution of personal-care aids. The company created some of the most widely used hair products (DOP shampoo, Imédia and Coloral dyes, and O'Cap gel for men), and it produced numerous skin-care products, cleansers, and cosmetics. Catering to an international clientele as early as 1912, Schueller learned quickly the value of manipulating new media to establish brand recognition and maximize profits. Among the first French businessmen to take out color advertisements in the press, he advertised on the radio in the 1920s and at the cinema in the 1930s, authored hygiene manuals devoted to young families, financed beauty contests, and created one of France's most popular lifestyle magazines, *La coiffure de Paris,* renamed *Votre beauté* in 1933.[39] Over the course of a century, L'Oréal was transformed from a small kitchen workshop into the world's largest producer of beauty products.[40] Perhaps the neighborhood pharmacist never stood a chance.

Of course, not every novice chemist founded a L'Oréal. Most manufacturers had to find viable retail outlets for their products, and many fabricators sold their goods in their own stores. Consumers continued to flock to the neighborhood pharmacy or to the local perfume shop to purchase soaps, powders, and creams. However, other manufacturers grew their businesses by peddling their wares as wholesalers. Consumers found these products on the shelves of three modern retailers: the department store, the beauty institute, and the hair salon.

The hallmark of the mid-nineteenth-century retailing revolution, the department store redefined retailer practices. The Bon Marché (1852), le Louvre (1855), the Bazar de l'Hôtel de Ville (1856), Au Printemps (1865), La Samaritaine (1869), and later, the Galeries Lafayette (1895) completely changed how producers and consumers conceptualized commodities. As early as the 1830s, dry goods stores called *magasins de nouveautés* began to group and sell items previously found at specialty shops. Unlike small retailers, these stores encouraged patrons to browse, allowed exchanges and reimbursements, and profited from high-volume turnover at low, fixed prices. Parisian department stores capitalized on the sales ingenuity of the *magasins de nouveautés,* but they also benefitted from changes in textile production, finance capitalism, Haussmanization, and transportation. Investors and industrialists made the huge emporia possible by absorbing start-up costs and stimulating new markets (like that of ready-to-wear clothing). Baron Haussmann's urban restructuring of Paris created grand boulevards that facilitated movement and paved the way for a bus and tram system that could carry customers and goods throughout the city and eventually into surrounding neighborhoods. Additionally, the railroad brought provincial shoppers into the metropolis and carried Paris to the provinces through the phenomenon of catalogue retailing.[41]

French department stores were not only inheritors of developments in retailing, but they also initiated change by enforcing cash-only policies, installing internal mail-order departments, placing salespeople in the service of customers, and creating opulent, pleasurable environments in which shopping became an experience rather than a duty. The historian Michael Miller has argued that these innovations fostered a "new concept of the bourgeois community" because stores like the Bon Marché, along with its catalogues, *agendas,* and trading cards, reinforced the values of an idealized class culture and exported those values from Paris to the provinces. Although the bourgeoisie's exclusive dominion over the department store is questionable, considering the store an imagined bourgeois community begins to explain how new merchant environments legitimized cosmetics use among middle-class women. As Miller points out, the Bon Marché, a store that catered to a predominantly Catholic and provincial clientele, added a perfume department in 1875 and incorporated cosmetics in its store and in its catalogues by 1900.[42] If a new bourgeois culture was indeed emerging with the department store, it was a culture that accepted, even embraced, beauty products.

The department store allowed women of all classes to envision themselves as part of a bourgeois world at the same time that it encouraged consumers to indulge in their most intimate, personal fantasies. Although middle-class women rubbed shoulders with shoppers and salespeople of other classes, and though critics worried that the sensory stimuli of store interiors would overwhelm feminine sensibilities, the department store nevertheless attracted respectable female shoppers. In fact, by replicating domestic interiors and maintaining constant masculine surveillance over both employees and customers, they provided women with an urban safe haven.[43] Through elaborate displays and a seemingly infinite supply of novelties, department stores seduced impressionable women at the same time that they provided them with a public forum for self-expression and self-performance.[44]

Beauty products played a crucial role in sustaining these fantasies. When department stores included cosmetics in their inventories, they rehabilitated them by welcoming the once reprehensible products into the metaphorical bourgeois home, allowing respectable women to guiltlessly purchase them alongside other goods commensurate with middle-class taste. Product selection was, however, a matter of individual discretion. Standing in front of the makeup counter or pouring over a department store *agenda* filled with images of the latest products, women could peruse the ever-expanding varieties of powders and rouges and imagine how they might look wearing them. Inside the store or absorbed in a catalogue, the matriarch, salesgirl, socialite, or provincial could imagine herself anew.

Although women could fantasize for free, their ability to actually purchase the products that enchanted them remained limited. During this period, women did increasingly gain access to their own discretionary incomes. Women comprised 34 percent of the French workforce in 1886, and half of the female population over age fifteen was employed in 1906. They were legally authorized to set up and maintain personal savings accounts in 1886; and, in 1907, married women were granted the right to use wages they earned without consulting husbands.[45] Yet, in 1908 an average box of powder cost 4.50 francs, and the typical Parisian workingwoman earned around 30 centimes an hour, or about 3 francs a day, for a ten-hour workday, which amounted to 15 francs a week for a fifty-hour workweek.[46] But even for women who could not afford to purchase cosmetics, the seduction of the decadently arranged department store displays encouraged virtual consumption. As Stephen Gundle has explained, cosmetics and "other goods that could be carried" were especially tantalizing because "they bore directly on personal identity, and promised the immediate realization of a transformation of the self into something different and better."[47] Inviting women to indulge, to dream, and to imagine themselves anew, department store displays of beauty products promoted the myth of democratized luxury.

Department stores offered consumers a fairly wide array of beauty aids; however, they did not yet provide the specialty products and services found in the new institutes and hair salons. The first beauty institutes functioned as public *cabinets de toilettes* for wealthy patrons, while salons promoted new fashions in hair care among the bourgeoisie. Both businesses featured a predominantly female clientele, and many boasted female proprietors and employees. Most importantly, institutes and hair salons brought private cleansing rituals into the domain of commerce and made public the respectable woman's pursuit of beauty.

Believing that women deserved more than mere creams and serums, Marie Valentin Le Brun opened France's first beauty institute on the place Vendôme in 1895. Catering exclusively to an elite and international clientele, Le Brun stocked her shelves with her own line of all-natural Klytia products and filled her institute with knowledgeable employees who pampered patrons with skin-care regimens, massages, manicures, and facials. The Société Athéna, the Institut médical des agents physiques, and the Institut scientifique de la beauté soon joined Le Brun's Klytia institute. These lavish institutes offered consultations with qualified aestheticians (another new profession), provided elaborate skin treatments, and employed novel procedures that could "correct facial imperfections." In 1912, the Australian-born Helena Rubinstein opened the first comprehensive, full-body institute in Paris. Rubinstein's institute offered the same goods and services as the others; however, it also incorporated spa elements like hydrotherapy and made available the newest scientific procedures including electrolysis and rudimentary plastic surgery.

Institutes provided women with new professional opportunities and introduced elite clients to unique services and products; however, fewer women visited or worked in institutes than patronized or labored in hair salons. Although men, notably Antoine, Marcel Grateau, Georges Dupuy, and Emile Long, were the most celebrated hairstylists of the day, the number of female clients and of women entering the hair profession increased dramatically in the first decades of the twentieth century. Paris supported 1,800 *salons mixtes* in 1889 but maintained 2,000 *salon de dames* alone by 1918. Similarly, whereas 10 percent of the profession was comprised by women in 1896, by 1946 women made up a majority, 54 percent, of all hairdressers.[48] Although women's professional opportunities remained limited (only 5,684 of the 60,709 "ouvriers and patrons" were women), they were regarded as "heads of enterprise" within the profession in 1911.[49]

These opportunities brought more women into the world of commerce and provided some petty bourgeois and working-class women with incomes of their own. This was especially the case during and immediately after the Great War, when women from the lower classes obtained quick training as apprentices in hair salons. Women employed in salons were encouraged, like saleswomen in department stores, to "look the part." Looking the part meant wearing the popular hairstyles, using the appropriate beauty products, and dressing and comporting oneself in a particular (i.e., bourgeois) fashion. Because workingwomen in the growing tertiary sector purchased creams and tonics to perform their professional roles, beauty products would become one of the first democratized luxury items.

Despite the participation of both sexes in the production, distribution, and consumption of aids and services, men and women fostered different relationships to the professionalization of beauty. As chemists, pharmacists, department-store owners, and elite hairdressers, men dominated the top sectors of the beauty industry, and they stood to profit most from the sale of new products. Male influence in the profession was especially pronounced in France, in part because French women were slower to enter the top echelons of the industry (especially when compared to their Anglo-American counterparts Harriet Hubbard Ayer, Helena Rubinstein, and their African American contemporary Madame C. J. Walker). Men did not, however, control all segments of the French beauty business because women increasingly entered the profession as hairdressers, institute proprietors, and even as product manufacturers and spokeswomen. Just as men did not maintain a monopoly over the production and sale of beauty, neither did women monopolize the consumption of aids and services. Women were much more likely to frequent salons and institutes and to buy personal-care items, but men continued to visit local barbers, and they purchased not only toothpastes and deodorants but also hair dyes and shaving creams.

Nevertheless, salon going quickly signaled a particular, gendered class status—bourgeois womanhood. Like the department store and the institute, the salon sold more than products and services; it also fostered sociability among women. Here patrons could admire shelves teeming with new products, peruse the latest editions of fashionable lifestyle magazines, converse with fellow clients or workers, or simply observe others as they partook in their own rituals of beautification. Having one's hair professionally cleansed and styled also provided women an easy, even enjoyable way to comply with contemporary hygiene initiatives. The salon made the toilette public and became an important site for making visible the middle-class woman's commitment to beauty. It provided, in Kathy Peiss's assessment, spaces of female mingling that "contributed substantially to modern definitions of femininity, to the growing emphasis on making and monitoring appearance, and to the centrality of commerce and consumption in women's lives." Like the beauty institute and the department store, the hair salon correlated respectable femininity with the pursuit of beauty, the liberty to consume, and the public performance of a female self.[50]

ADVERTISING BEAUTY

Just as new merchant environments publicized the products and practices of beautification, advertisements brought feminine beauty secrets into plain sight. Yet French businesses were slow to adopt modern marketing techniques. For one thing, French firms encountered economic and cultural constraints. Advertising was expensive because the press demanded high rates that varied depending upon a firm's seniority, the product for sale, and the regularity of advertising orders. Moreover, few French firms mass-produced goods, which translated into fewer brand names and a lower demand for regional and national ad campaigns. Advertising also threatened the interests of middlemen (especially traveling salesmen) who conventionally facilitated transactions between producers and retailers.[51] In addition to these economic limitations, French firms encountered a public hostile or (at best) indifferent to ads. The number of "quack pharmaceutical" ads that proliferated in the nineteenth-century press, for example, created the general impression that publicity was untrustworthy, manipulative, or insincere. Not only did consumers mistrust ads, but some of them also believed that advertising costs were passed onto them. Conversely, many commercial organizations rejected ads because they thought that structured advertising "impinged upon retailer independence."[52]

In the 1880s and 1890s, three important developments facilitated the modernization of French advertising: first, technological advancements in ink and print making permitted the cheaper reproduction of color images; second, new laws eased state control over the media; and third, city councils allowed commercial rental of city-owned walls. Although lacking the psychological depth and technical sophistication found in campaigns launched by Anglo-American and German competitors, French beauty firms began to invest in print and poster advertisements.[53] Advertisements legitimized cosmetics use by acquainting consumers with beauty brands and testifying to product safety and efficacy, while retailers employed new advertising strategies to create a middle-class market for beauty products.

As the volume of beauty products entering the market increased, firms learned to distinguish their brand from those of competitors. Firms competed for space in *vitrines,* merchant window displays. The *vitrine* offered a visually stimulating canvas that used lighting and the artistic staging of goods to "create desire and to sell."[54] Firms wanted their products displayed in these windows and increasingly created unique names and distinctive packages for their products. One strategy that firms used to distinguish their brand was to give their products names that had aristocratic associations. This strategy, which would have been unthinkable in the early nineteenth century, became quite commonplace in the middle years of the Third Republic. At this time, royal couples were revered as popular celebrities, and nostalgia for France's diminishing aristocracy, which had reached an all-time high, sharpened the public's desire for luxury.[55] Responding to this demand for extravagance, many manufacturers wrapped aids in elegant packaging. The casing for Fleur de Bouquet not only acted as a decorative container for the product but could be featured in a *vitrine* display, in the *cabinet de toilette,* or even in the boudoir as an objet d'art.[56] On display, the bottle associated retailers with high quality, consumers with good taste, and both with France's glorious aristocratic past. Collecting several of these decorative containers, moreover, enabled the consumer to surround herself with her own personal miniature world of luxury and to cast herself as an inheritor of French grandeur.

More than any other late-nineteenth-century advertising strategy, periodical advertisements correlated the consumption of health and beauty aids with respectable bourgeois femininity. At a time when ineffective health and beauty aids posed as genuine remedies by making fraudulent claims, advertisers had to work hard to prove the efficacy of legitimate products. One of the ways that they did this was by explicitly spelling out a product's scientific merits and health benefits. Language and tone were especially important aspects of these ads because they created a context for the commodity, defined the good's intended consumer, and established the manufacturer's credibility. Beauty ads "spoke" in a variety of scripted voices, the anonymous voice and the voice of the professional being the most prominent among them.[57] Ads relied on reason, evidence, testimony, and modeling to convince consumers that purchasing a product necessitated an informed choice at the same time that they addressed their appeals to certain types of consumer—the aging matron, the dutiful wife, and the youthful coquette. While a rational conception of beauty implicitly advocated a scientific approach to self-care that conveniently echoed the manuals authored by health-care professionals, the evocation of consumer types acknowledged differences among women and reinforced the belief that beauty was every woman's responsibility.

Evoking the anonymous voice, which personally appealed to the consumer by posing as an objective but informed confidante, was a pervasive strategy within periodical advertisements. In a matter-of-fact tone, the anonymous voice highlighted the product, explained its utility and effects, and influenced beauty behaviors. A 1909 Crème Simon ad for soap and powder demonstrates this strategy.[58] The ad displays the two products and two women at either side of the page. The women appear to have no relation to one another or to the commodities shown. Located at the bottom of the page, detached from both the products and the models, the text assures readers that Simon aids were "marvelous for the health and beauty of the skin." It then warns consumers to accept "no imitations or substitutions." Likewise, an ad for Lait des Alpes features a woman at her toilette smiling into her mirror as she applies the product.[59] Although the text framing the scene promises that Lait des Alpes is superior to "all creams and rice powders," it is not clear that the woman in the ad is advancing the claim. The Crème Simon ad and the one for Lait des Alpes both address the mature woman through an anonymous, authoritative voice, and they each do so to demonstrate, in a seemingly objective manner, that personal hygiene signifies true feminine beauty at any age. Marketed as a "marvelous product for the health and beauty of the skin," the Crème Simon ad indicates that hygiene precedes beauty and that beauty derives from good health. Although the Lait des Alpes ad is less explicit, the model's glowing skin, orderly hair arrangement, and organized toilette table all imply that cleanliness is a priority for her as well. Correlating beauty with hygiene, the anonymous voice in these ads promotes feminine self-care as a beneficial form of woman's work.

The most common form of advertisement to speak with an anonymous voice was the testimonial. Often disguised as press articles, these "advertorials" blurred the line between publicity and reportage. A. Autard exemplified how some firms adopted this strategy. One of its wrinkle cream ads provides before-and-after images of a fifty-eight-year-old woman surrounded by text claiming that she was "completely transformed" by Autard cream.[60] The cream, the ad promises, could make people between fifty and sixty years old look as they did in their early thirties. Although the ad focuses on aging rather than cleanliness, the underlying message (as well as the need for the product) relates to broader concerns about disease and depopulation. In 1908, the French remained concerned about limited population growth at the same time that the nation engaged in imperial struggles and witnessed Germany's increasing demands for relevance in the world stage. The ad, in many ways, can be read as a metaphor for these anxieties. Hygiene and beauty, united here in the image of the aging woman, signals the decaying nation: just as France required babies to rejuvenate the nation, women needed Autard wrinkle cream to revitalize the self. It was woman's duty to repopulate the aging nation and to restore both her body and France to its youthful splendor.

In addition to posing as objective counsel, "woman in the mirror" advertisements also showed women using beauty aids. Numerous ads used this scenario to demonstrate appropriate product application and to give products meaning. "Women in the mirror" ads generally featured adult women in the prime of life. Posed in one of two ways—either looking at the viewer or absorbed in her own reflected image—these women appear self-possessed.

Nover's 1900 ad for la parfumerie IDEA shows a woman, her back facing the viewer, looking through her mirror and holding a perfume bottle.[61] Dressed in bourgeois fashion, the woman is surrounded by other beauty products. Though interrupted from her own self-care regimen, she graciously smiles through the mirror at the viewer, bringing the interloper into her confidence. More sororial than seductive, the image nonetheless recalls the intimate tone of Dr. Schultz's manual. Both depict a respectable woman engaged in a personal, private practice to reaffirm woman's commitment to beauty work.

Other advertisements implied that women could be "caught in the act" of beautification. A Gellé Frères ad featured a woman applying powder in front of two male onlookers seated in her *cabinet de toilette.*[62] Seemingly engrossed in conversation with the men, the woman appears totally oblivious to the viewer. Unlike the "woman in the mirror ad" described above, this image clearly situates the woman as the object of two gazes—the onlookers in the scene and the advertisement viewer. In so doing, it blatantly contradicts the image of the sanitized cabinet endorsed by hygiene manuals. In a different vein but containing a similar message, an 1893 ad for Felix Potin Parfumerie featured an elegantly coiffed woman in evening dress applying her powder while peering into her hand-held mirror.[63] Completely absorbed in her own image the woman seems unaware or unconcerned that she is on display. Moreover, her body is intentionally positioned away from the viewer at a forty-five-degree angle. Women in the mirror either invited onlookers into the cabinet with them, or, like this one, they appeared altogether oblivious to the fact that anyone was looking at them at all. In the first scenario, the woman knowingly performs for her audience; in the second, she submits fully to pleasuring herself. In both cases, however, woman cast herself in the image of desire; she forfeits her privacy in the first instance, her propriety in the second, to transform her body into the object of the mass gaze.

Caught-in-the-act posters, like Jules Chéret's famous ad for Cosmydor soap (fig. 1.1), were even more playful and eye-catching. Calling attention to the corseted model's rosy cheeks and come-hither glance, the colorful poster flagrantly insinuates the model's sexuality. It is no small irony, then (and we may even envision the artist's own playful wink), that this impish woman is selling the purest of all artificial aids—soap! Beauty companies employed art nouveau artists, like Chéret, who emphasized the sensuality of their subjects because this art form was stylistically compatible with an industry whose products were in constant contact with the female body.[64]

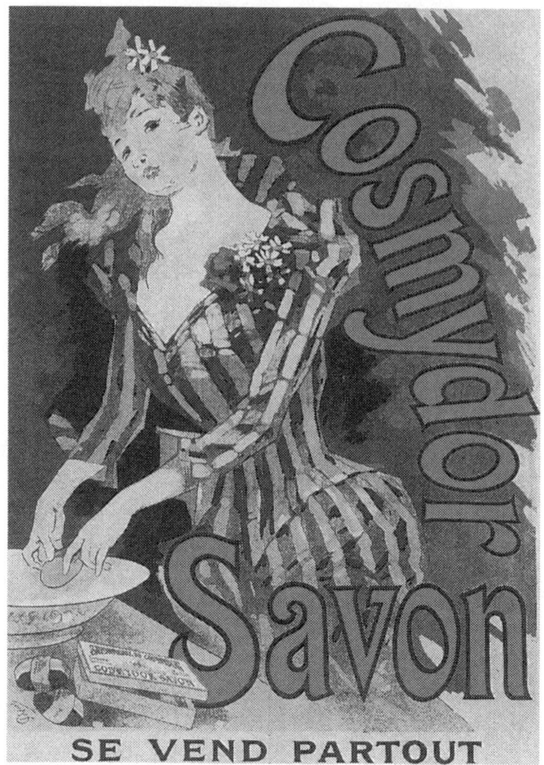

Fig. 1.1. Jules Chéret, Cosmydor savon, se vend partout. Paris, impr., Chaix, 1891.

The performative quality of making up was reinforced by advertisements featuring actresses, models, and women of the *monde élégant*. The high-end Parfumerie Charlet marketed itself exclusively to "women of quality." An 1893 ad for the product shows a typical "woman-in-the-mirror" scenario; however, this woman's class status is conveyed by her Louis XV dressing table, her evening gown (and the amount of décolletage that it revealed), and her intricately crafted hand mirror. The message of the ad was twofold—viewers who could not afford such luxuries could not afford Charlet, and using Charlet was a marker of social distinction. These messages, however, did not preclude viewers from imagining themselves as able to afford the product or as belonging to the society that it represented. Actresses frequently endorsed beauty products: Berthe Séon signed testimonials for Adair's self-care products and services, and, in 1905, the Comédie-Française actress Mlle. Bardet deemed Le Perle powder "remarkable." Sarah Bernhardt is depicted in Jules Chéret's famous 1890 ad for La Diaphane generously powdering her face as she prepares for either an evening out or a stage performance (fig. 1.2).[65] Here Bernhardt epitomized the art nouveau look—decoratively adorned, her pose emphasized her sinewy body and augmented her palpable carefree pleasure. Chéret depicted the actress not only as a seductive temptress but also as a woman who basked in self-care. Moreover, this image played on the average woman's fantasy of glamour—on the one hand, Sarah Bernhardt applying powder, one of the most widely used cosmetics of the time, was not so unlike the bourgeois housewife applying powder before spending a day about town; on the other, viewers could imagine themselves covering their own bodies with powder to create themselves in the image of their favorite actress.

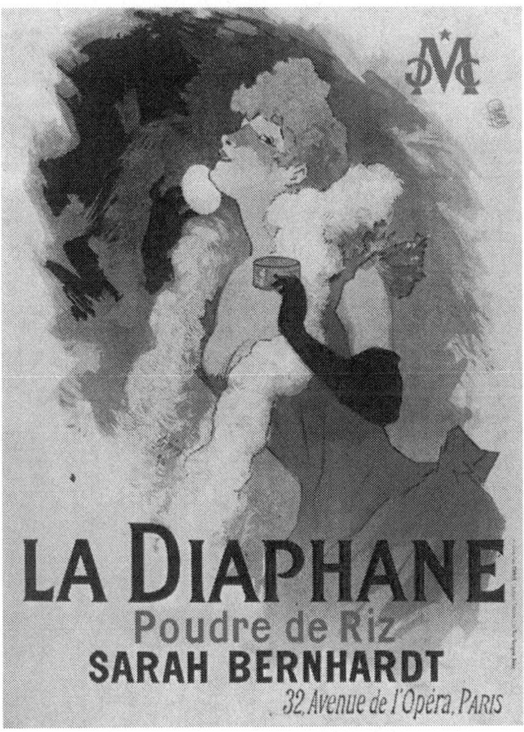

Fig. 1.2. Jules Chéret. La Diaphane: Poudre de riz, Sarah Bernhardt. Paris, impr. Chaix, 1890.

Although mass-media publicity was not yet ingrained in France, by the fin de siècle publicists were learning how to cultivate public opinion and how to target audiences. Beauty advertisements identified female consumers as potential purchasers, but they also imagined them as bodies that could be, in Margaret Beetham's words, "constructed by and through commodities."[66] In 1898, for example, Japhet depicted a hypersexualized, Venus-like woman emerging naked from a bowl of Eau Tonique Dicquemare, a product intended to rejuvenate the hair. Surrounded on the left by her flowing hair, which conceals her face and her genitals while leaving the rest of her body exposed, this Venus applies the tonic overhead with her right arm. The ad's message: Dicquemare's Venus was born from neither the gods nor the theater, but from a little bottle of magical hair tonic. Hence advertising images were not accidental or arbitrary but, rather, carefully conceived strategies deployed to stimulate consumer desire.

At the fin de siècle, beauty advertisements became a privileged site for the negotiation of feminine identity. Advertisements depicted feminine beauty as an ideal achievable through vigilant effort. They portrayed the female body as fragmented, inadequate, and incomplete and implied that women could become whole and desirable through diligent work. Ads linked a middle-class woman's identity to her physical appearance and made clear that the French woman was a woman on view. As a public spectacle, the middle-class woman engaged in the work of beauty and made personal appearance a top priority.

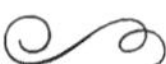

Health-care professionals, beauty businesses, and advertisers legitimized the middle-class woman's use of artifice by linking hygiene with aesthetics. Hygienists and physicians argued that through corporeal upkeep women could serve family and nation by curtailing the spread of disease and solving the problem of depopulation. To this end, they promoted beauty work as an essential component of bourgeois womanhood. Advances in the fabrication of less-toxic aids also shaped the public's increasingly tolerant attitude toward artifice. By eliminating the health risks associated with previously available products, manufacturers provided the respectable woman with indispensible tools for safely achieving good hygiene while augmenting her corporeal beauty. That these new products were sold in the hallmarks of middle-class commerce—the department store, the beauty institute, and the hair salon—only underscored their growing social acceptance.

Ironically, by making beauty work essential to middle-class womanhood, health-care professionals, beauty businesses, and advertisements challenged two important bourgeois convictions: one that understood artifice as a marker of moral corruption; and another that suggested that virtuous women were simply born beautiful. Certainly, these groups endorsed the use of creams, powders, and even visible cosmetics to serve their own agendas. Health-care professionals envisioned beauty aids as valuable weapons in the war against germs and disease, while firms and ads stood to profit financially from their sale. However, by characterizing artificial products as inoffensive, safe, and necessary, these groups divested artifice of its dubious reputation and legitimized its use. At the same time, they also unmasked the work that went into making women beautiful. Implicit in the promotion of artifice was the belief that women's bodies were naturally flawed and in need of augmentation. To correct corporeal imperfections, middle-class women were expected to commit fully to beauty work, for beauty was not only woman's desire; it was also her duty.

2

The Work of Beauty

Woman's power resides in her beauty.
—Vicomtesse de Nacla, *Le boudoir: Conseils d'élégance,* 1896

In her *Illustrated Encyclopedia of Elegance: The Hygiene of Beauty* (1892), Mme. Charles Boeswilwald (writing under the pseudonym André-Valdès) confided to her readers that feminine beauty constituted a process of serious and constant learning. Boeswilwald shared with health-care professionals concerns about hygiene and the belief that personal cleanliness was a precursor to good health. Unlike them, however, she did not use the language of science to abstract the female body from her discussions of self-care. In a straightforward manner, she explicitly linked health and beauty to female sexuality.[1] The first chapter of her "practical manual," coyly entitled "Morality and the *Necessity* of Coquetry,"[2] spoke directly to the respectable bourgeois. "So often I hear married women say with touching simplicity 'Oh me, I no longer need to be a coquette, I am married, and I no longer need to be pleasing, moreover, I love my husband.' Oh! How you deceive yourself, madam! You no longer need to please because you are married? Au contraire, this is the moment to be a coquette and to please, if you wish to keep the heart that you have conquered!"[3] Although she correlated coquetry with woman's duty to please and to be pleasing to the opposite sex, Boeswilwald nevertheless acknowledged woman's seductive power and, in so doing, exposed the complicated relationship between female sexuality and middle-class womanhood.[4]

Indeed, Boeswilwald's attempt to reconcile morality with coquetry spoke to a broader cultural debate regarding the problem of female respectability. According to nineteenth-century gender ideology, bourgeois women were biologically incapable of sexual feeling, they found comfort in the protected spaces of domestic life, and they acted always as selfless martyrs, suppressing their own desires to the needs of family and class. Discursively produced in republican rhetoric, religious lessons, and domestic novels, to name but a few sources, this ideology established a rigid template for female respectability that, despite its apparent authoritative certainty, was riddled with contradiction. For example, even if she engaged in intercourse only reluctantly—tolerating it as a necessary, if disagreeable duty—the demands placed upon the married woman trapped her in a double bind: on the one hand, she was expected to deny herself gratification; on the other, she was advised to use sex to, in Boeswilwald's words, "keep the heart that [she had] conquered." Casting the middle-class woman in the role of coquette, Boeswilwald linked a wife's pursuit of beauty to her duty to please and to give sexual pleasure. In so doing, she opened a space for respectable women to imagine and even to assert sexual agency.

Boeswilwald was not alone in her endeavor to redefine female respectability in the late nineteenth century. This chapter examines how the Nineteenth-Century Venus, the Grand Coquette, and the Beauty Countess, models of womanhood generated in art and literature, the woman's periodical, and the self-help manual, respectively, participated in this same work. Art historians, literary critics, and historians of gender have generally read these well-known figures independent of one another; however, considering them together and within the context of France's emergent commercial beauty culture shows the complex processes through which these media helped produce the feminine. In the works of Édouard Manet and Émile Zola, the Nineteenth-Century Venus seductively coupled beauty with desire to challenge the notion that women were devoid of sexual feeling. Peppering their pages with glamorous images of the Grand Coquette, periodicals produced an aspirational model of beauty for ordinary women to emulate. In their advice manuals and breviaries, Beauty Countesses condoned woman's use of artifice and legitimized her pursuit of beauty by characterizing beautification as a valid and enjoyable form of woman's work. Ultimately, the hypothetical models of womanhood that emerged within these cultural media proposed alternatives to bourgeois respectability at the same time that they expanded the range of acceptable social roles available to middle-class French women.

THE NINETEENTH-CENTURY VENUS

For centuries Venus, the mythical goddess of love, beauty, and fecundity, has symbolized man's ultimate sexual fantasy. Originally appreciated for her capacity to embody feminine charm and grace, by the third century BCE, Venus signified seduction, sexual desire, and carnal indulgence. It was this second iteration that the impressionist artist Édouard Manet and naturalist writer Émile Zola evoked in their renderings of Olympia and Nana. Defined by her raw sexual power and driven by her own insatiable desires, the Nineteenth-Century Venus, as she emerged through these cultural productions, titillated and scandalized. Moreover, presented as objects and agents of both the commercial and sexual marketplace of middle-class Paris, Manet's and Zola's fictional working-class prostitutes exemplified one of the many unpredictable ways that bourgeois respectability was constructed through male-generated images of sexually promiscuous, class-indeterminate women.

From the moment of its début at the 1865 salon, Manet's painting of an enigmatic odalisque, titled *Olympia,* fueled social anxieties (fig. 2.1).[5] Based loosely on Titian's sixteenth-century *Venus of Urbino,* Manet's reclining nude recalled the overt eroticism of her enchanting predecessor. But whereas the soft flesh, full lip, and curved eye of Titian's Venus welcomed viewers, the angular body, overwrought pose, and clinched mouth of Manet's Olympia reviled them. The critic and onlooker Paul de Saint-Victor described "the crowd

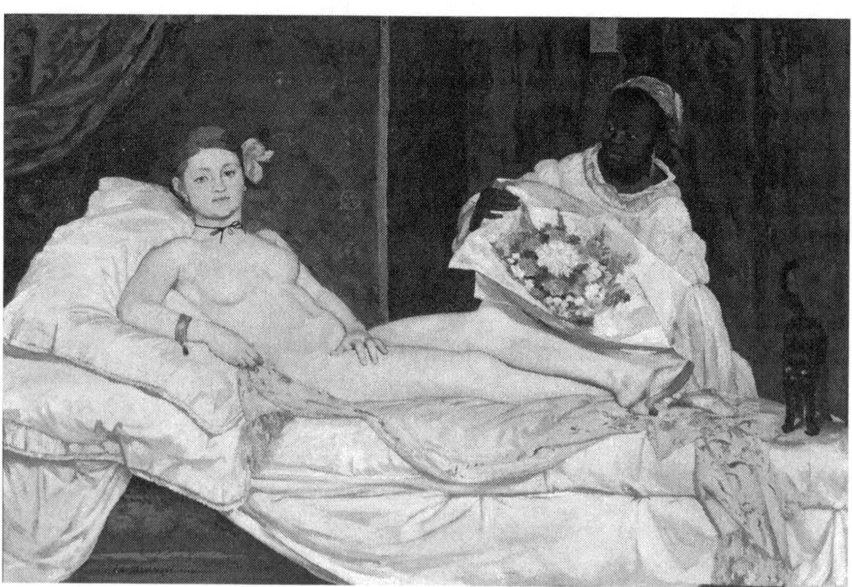

Fig. 2.1. Édouard Manet, *Olympia,* 1865, © RMN-Grand Palais / Art Resource, NY.

thronging in front of the putrefied *Olympia* as if it were at a morgue."[6] Unable to decipher its meaning, male viewers found Olympia's unwavering, vacant, kohl-rimmed stare particularly unsettling.[7] Discomfort within the crowd arose not only from Olympia's challenging gaze but also from her corpse-like body.[8] The stiff alignment of her left arm, which effectively covered over (and by extension denied access to) her sex, the empty gaze that refused to engage, and the yellowing flesh whose sickly paleness suggested bodily decay fascinated onlookers, who pressed "up to the picture as if to a hanged man."[9] Thus rather than inflame masculine desire, as the *Urbino* Venus had, Olympia challenged it. Like her predecessors, Olympia invited men to openly gaze upon the nude female body; however, because her body was neither classically beautiful nor appropriately submissive, she deprived men the carnal pleasure derived from the privilege of voyeuristic looking.

Perhaps even more disquieting than Olympia's frankness was that she was not an allegorical representation but an identifiable, living woman—the model and artist Victorine Meurent. A well-known workingwoman with ties to bourgeois bohemia and who posed as a high-class courtesan, in representation as in reality, Meurent blurred class distinctions. Manet further capitalized on Meurent's classlessness by calling his portrait *Olympia,* a name commonly taken by ordinary Parisian prostitutes. Choosing this name, Manet not only blatantly positioned his subject at the intersection of sex and commerce but also stripped away any reference to the mythical by transforming the immortal Venus into an embodied, erotic mass commodity. Manet's choice of subject matter was not particularly innovative for the 1860s, as prostitutes were regularly featured in the literature, gossip books, and sociological texts of the decade.[10] What was remarkable, as T. J. Clark has pointed out, was that of the more than seventy published accounts dedicated to *Olympia* in 1865, only a handful referenced prostitution.[11] This omission leads Clark to assert that it was not Olympia's sexuality itself that troubled viewers but the fact that Manet gave his "female subject a particular sexuality as opposed to a general one."[12] Locating sexuality in the nude body of his real-life subject, rather than in an abstract figure, Manet challenged an uncritical reading of the prostitute as merely an anonymous object of masculine desire. Understood in this way, perhaps it was less Olympia's apparent lifelessness and more her too lifelike connection to her sex and to her sexuality that viewers found so disconcerting.

Whether they came to gawk, to chuckle, to ridicule, or simply to see what all of the fuss was about, large crowds of spectators, male and female, and by contemporary accounts, representing all social classes, flocked to the salon to see *Olympia*. As A. Bonnin recorded in his article for *La France*, "Each day [*Olympia*] is surrounded by a crowd of visitors, and in this constantly changing group, reflections and observations are made out loud which spare the picture no part of the truth." He went on to explain, "Some people are delighted, they think it a joke that they want to look as if they understood; others observe the thing seriously and show their neighbor, here a well-placed tone, there a hand which is improper, but nicely painted; finally one sees painters whose work was rejected by the salon jury this year—and there is proof that they do exist—standing in front of the picture, beside themselves with spite and indignation."[13]

Fifteen years after *Olympia* scandalized the city, another even more seductive and more problematic prostitute captured the Parisian imagination. Weaving an intricate social commentary through the simultaneous embodiment and disembodiment of his doomed heroine, the oversexed Nana Coupeau, Émile Zola explored female sexual power in his 1880 novel *Nana*. The novel, an instant best seller that went through more than fifty printings in the first weeks after its publication, recounts the story of a mediocre stage performer who uses her sexual allure to become a favored Parisian paramour.[14] As an actress and courtesan, Nana's identity resides in her dual status as a producer of sexual fantasy and as an erotic commodity. Nana earns her living and derives both her market and her social value exclusively from her ability to produce herself as an exchangeable good for sale. Yet Nana represents more than a mere object for exchange; she also personifies the overstimulated consumer.[15] Abandoning herself completely to the pursuit of pleasure, Nana spends her earnings recklessly on rich foods, useless trinkets, and gaudy fashions. Her escapades as well as her deft navigation of Paris's commercial and sexual marketplaces reveal a woman not simply shopping, but a glutton who cannot, at any cost, deprive herself of carnal or material pleasures. In the figure of Zola's Nana, then, the Nineteenth-Century Venus emerged as a vexing vixen who rendered female desire for sex or for things both a social problem and an indisputable reality.

Zola explores the problem posed by woman's unregulated desire in the opening scene of the novel, in which Nana makes her much-anticipated stage début as the Blonde Venus. Initially, she offends the audience with her "voix vinaigrée," but she soon wins it over when she laughs heartily at her own lack of skill.[16] Though Nana unabashedly admitted "that she had no talent at all," she uses her body language to tell onlookers "that it did not matter because she had something else" (18). Nana's playfulness disarms her audience, but it is the seductive display of her nude body in the second scene that enables her to conquer it completely. "The crowd was thrilled. Nana was naked, naked and unashamed, serenely confident in the irresistible power of her young flesh.... Covered by a simple veil, her whole body could be seen, or imagined, by everyone through the diaphanous, white, frothy gauze" (31–32). The enraptured spectator submits, intoxicated by Nana's body, the music, and the smell of warm flesh. In an erotic euphoria, the scene culminates with Nana "facing the ecstatic audience of fifteen hundred people, that was crammed together and overcome by the exhausted and nervous prostration, inevitable at the end of any show, Nana's body, as smooth and white as marble, was all-conquering, her sexuality powerful enough to destroy all these people and to remain unscathed" (34).

When Nana appears as Venus, draped in nothing but her hair, a thin veil, and a veneer of cosmetics, she shamelessly uses her beautiful body to seduce her audience. Here, at the height of her fame, Nana—plump and in the prime of life—starkly contrasts with Manet's sickly, sallow Olympia. Yet by the end of the novel, Nana, too, is in physical decline, paying the price for her hedonism. The narrative of unchecked feminine passion links both women to one another and to their profession. Both Nana and Olympia derive their sexual power from consciously creating themselves as objects of male desire. As is evident in Nana's every flick of the hip, every sideways glance that ends in a suggestive wink, and in Olympia's unwavering gaze and her suggestively dangling shoe, these Venuses act as gatekeepers for the carnal underworld of Paris. As such, they invite bourgeois men into their world not as masters but as powerless servants of their own perverted fantasies.

Zola establishes the important role that cosmetics play in the prostitute's acquisition of this power. Following her performance as the Blonde Venus, Nana retreats backstage, where her most ardent admirer, Count Muffat, ogles her. Muffat is suffocated by "the sharp scent of toilet water and soap drifting from the dressing-rooms mixed with the pestilential odor of human breath" and is mesmerized by "des senteurs de femmes," the musky odor of makeup blended with the scent of human hair (152). He fetishizes the objects in Nana's *cabinet de toilette,* fixating on "a white marble dressing table filled with cut-glass containers and bottles of creams, perfumes, and face powders. The count went to the mirror and saw that his own face was very red, with small beads of perspiration on his forehead; he lowered his eyes, walked over to the dressing-table, and seemed for a moment to be absorbed in the wash basin filled with soapy water, the scattered little ivory implements, and wet sponges" (153). Confronted with the tools of Nana's trade, the props that enable her to transform herself into the Venus, Muffat can no longer mask his arousal. Forced to lower his eyes, with red face and perspiring brow, the count literally surrenders the gaze and concedes Nana's power over him.

Ignoring Muffat and her other male devotees, Nana begins powdering her face and arms before smearing her body with cold cream and grease paint. In complete command of her audience, she picks up "the hare's paw and, with great concentration, was lightly rubbing it across her skin, arching her body over the dressing table so that her white trousers stretched tightly over her plump bottom with the little tag of her shift showing above" (160). The spectators, who until now chatted easily with the performer, observe a respectful silence. After coating herself in a film of rice powder, "she became very serious; she was about to apply her rouge. Once again, holding her face next to the mirror, she dipped her finger into a jar and rubbed rouge under her eyes, spreading it gently along her temples" (160). As Nana carefully prepares her body for the next scene, Muffat watches in horror and in ecstasy: "She dipped the brush into a jar of mascara, and with her nose pressed against the mirror; she closed her left eye and stroked it delicately between her lashes." Muffat, despite his efforts, "could not remove his eyes from this face" (162–63).

In this scene, Nana's beauty cabinet sets the stage for Muffat's seduction. Lured into the private performance by the "sharp scent of toilette water," he views the cabinet/theater through "cut-glass containers and bottles of creams, perfumes and face powders." Slathering on grease paints, arching her body over her dressing table to cover it with powder, and rhythmically massaging her temples with rogue, Nana's toilette mimics sexual play. Muffat's attention focuses on a jar of mascara, but it is not until the mascara brush passed over Nana's second eye, making her look "overcome with desire," that the count acknowledged Nana's power over him. The two "broad streaks of rouge on her lips" prove Muffat's undoing as he submits completely to the "perversions of powders and rouges" (162–63).

Zola's Muffat was not the only man seduced by the "perversions of powders and rouges." Intrigued by the courtesan's hypnotic toilette, Manet submitted his own portrait of *Nana* (fig. 2.2) to the 1877 salon. Completed two years before Zola's novel was serialized in *Le Voltaire,* critics debate the extent

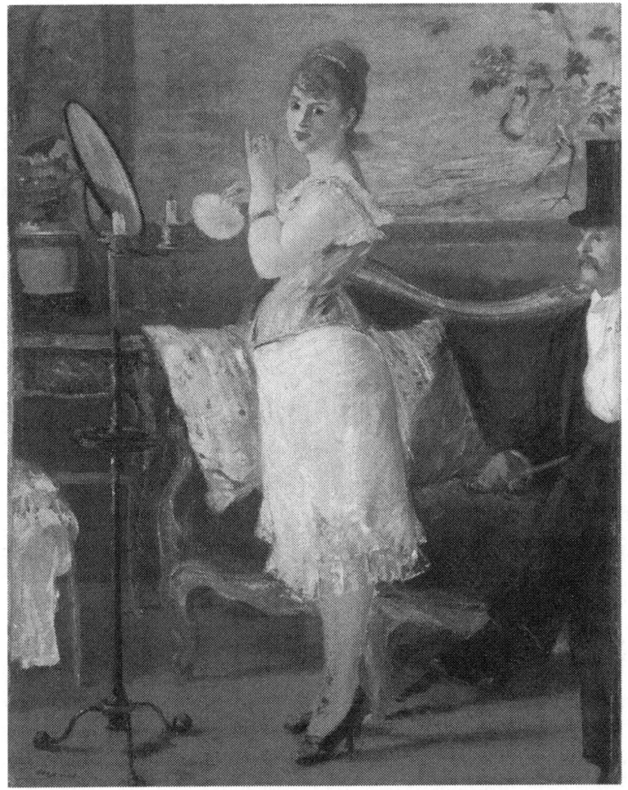

Fig. 2.2. Édouard Manet, *Nana,* 1877, bpk, Berlin / Hamburger Kunsthalle / Elke Walford / Art Resource, NY.

to which Manet's Nana was related to the author's. Although Zola's Nana may not have been fully realized in 1877—she had been introduced in *L'assommoir* (1877) as a struggling street urchin—Zola already mapped out her character in his notes for the 1880 novel. Nana, he decided, would be "nothing but flesh, but flesh in all its beauty." Manet's portrait, like Zola's scene above, features Nana's transformation into the Blonde Venus. Devoid of Olympia's insolence, Manet's Nana (embodied by the actress Henriette Hauser) flirtatiously welcomes the viewer. As Carol Armstrong explains, Nana gave what Olympia denied.[17] Manet's impish Nana basks in the glow of youth and delights in exciting men's passions. She makes no effort to conceal her powder puff or to cover over her partially exposed figure. She is also unconcerned by the male admirer (presumably Muffat), who, although positioned discreetly in the slightly cropped edge of the composition, attracts attention by openly staring at Nana's ample derriere. Aware that she is always an object on view, a human spectacle, Nana as depicted by both Manet and Zola turns even the most banal process of making up into a riveting erotic performance.

Like Manet, Zola recognizes that Nana's sexual power derives in part from the prostitute's self-love. Disrobing in her boudoir, Nana is overcome by her own unbridled passions. Nana stands in front of her mirror as, unbeknownst to her, Muffat looks on. "One of Nana's pleasures was undressing in front of her wardrobe where she could see her whole body in the mirror" (235). Completely nude, she contemplates "her satiny smooth skin, the flowing curves of her waist" (du satin de sa peau et de la ligne souple de sa taille [235]). Zola confides that Nana has made a habit of admiring her nudity and that she is frequently engrossed in acts of "*amour d'elle-même*" (self-love [235]). Recounted from Nana's viewpoint, the scene empowers the heroine, who, like her male admirers, derives satisfaction from looking at and possessing the prostitute's body.[18]

Not far into the scene, however, Zola shifts the narrative perspective to Muffat, and it is through his eyes that Nana's performance unfolds. Initially troubled by the way that she inspects her "torse de Vénus" (Venus-like torso) and how her hand lingers over her breasts and thighs, Muffat becomes aroused when she begins swaying and rolling her hips like an Egyptian belly dancer (237). He watches intently, simultaneously frightened by her bestial eroticism and repulsed by his own involuntary reaction to it. Nana, on the other hand, extorts a voluptuous laugh as she follows the reflection of her body thrusting and pulsating in the mirror. Nana's *plaisir solitaire* climaxes when, after fondling her breasts convulsively, "her lips breathed desire greedily over herself; she pursed [her lips] and placed a long kiss beside her armpit, laughing at the other Nana who was also kissing herself in the mirror" (239).

Nana's autoerotic performance signifies a power play inasmuch as it enables her to reclaim a body that lovers have attempted to colonize and to claim as their own. It is ironic that she achieves self-possession by using her body in the same manner as her lovers—as a fetishistic plaything. In front of the mirror, Nana co-opts the objectifying male gaze, and, in so doing, she challenges what Emily Apter has called "the erotic conditions of mastery" that confer her sex-object status.[19] Moreover, by taking pleasure in her own sexual play, Nana openly acknowledges woman's capacity for sexual feeling.

Nana's looking glass does more than reflect her subversive behavior; it positions readers in the text in such a way that they can only understand the prostitute's body itself as a mirror for social reflection. Confronted with woman's sexuality, Muffat "realized the disastrous effects of evil, [as] he saw the disorder caused by this festering wound, he himself would be poisoned, his family destroyed, a whole part of society would break up and collapse" (238). By linking Nana's narcissistic self-love with Muffat's hypocritical self-loathing, Zola echoed contemporary attitudes that linked feminine deviance with social malaise. Nana, however, was not solely responsible for the havoc she wrought—the Muffats of the world, driven to madness by their own complicity in the prostitute's sexual transgressions, were also implicated in her crimes. Like Olympia before her, Nana dared the viewer to see himself through her eyes, to recognize in himself that which he found most repulsive in her.

Although long venerated in the world of high art as a symbol of feminine grace, the Venus of Roman mythology was not only a martyr to love who could turn sexual vice into virtue, but also the pleasure-seeking goddess of prostitutes, whose Latin name meant, literally, "sexual desire." Manet and Zola played on this iteration to show how feminine sexuality was constructed as a problem in the nineteenth century.[20] Rife with contradictions, the Nineteenth-Century Venus offered a model of female sexual power that was simultaneously titillating and threatening. As sexually available purveyors of pleasure, Olympia and Nana indulged male fantasies at the same time that they exposed how middle-class morality could be produced through the image and behavior of the sexually promiscuous woman. On the one hand, forecasting woman's fall into depravity, the corpse-like Olympia and hedonistic Nana upheld class-based assumptions regarding the working-class woman. Unlike her virtuous middle-class counterpart, the workingwoman was closer to sex and in need of moral direction. In the guise of the prostitute, then, the Nineteenth-Century Venus operated as a cautionary tale that put middle- and working-class women firmly in their place.

On the other hand, in their depictions of Nana's metamorphosis into the Blonde Venus, Manet and Zola inadvertently offered respectable women a model for harnessing sexual power. By illuminating the secrets of her trade—her clothing, her cosmetics, her furnishings, her behaviors—Manet and Zola exposed Nana not as an ephemeral goddess, but as a carefully constructed agent of desire. Nana's sexual power emerged in part from her cosmetic manipulation of the female body. Through the sensual application of beauty products, Nana transformed and sexualized the female body. A peripheral figure, the pathologically sex-crazed working-class prostitute represented all that a respectable woman could not be: déclassé, carnal, degenerate. However, as respectable women increasingly engaged in beauty work, they could learn from Nana's example the sexual perils and rewards such work offered. Thus it was not only as masculine sex object but also as model of female behavior that the Nineteenth-Century Venus played her most subversive role.

THE GRAND COQUETTE

Men were the primary producers of the Nineteenth-Century Venus; however, fin-de-siècle Grand Coquettes emerged from the collaborative efforts of men and women employed by the feminine press. The nineteenth-century press painted the mercurial coquette as an enchanting marvel and a bewitching menace. Like the Venus, the coquette also offered an alternative to respectable womanhood. She privileged self-gratification over feminine duty, and her inclination toward indulgence revealed itself not only in an unwillingness to accept her domestic role but also in a voracious desire for consumer goods. The commercial marketplace, particularly that segment devoted to beauty and fashion, legitimized the coquette's pursuit of pleasure at the same time that it transformed her into a prepackaged, consumable commodity. Embodied by stunning socialites, alluring actresses, and notorious courtesans, the Grand Coquette made a public spectacle of feminine beauty and ambition. In the process, she promoted a glamorous model of womanhood that middle-class women sought to emulate. Unlike the Nineteenth-Century Venus, whose raw sexuality overtly threatened the status quo, the Grand Coquette's challenge was subtler and therefore more adaptable to the middle-class lifestyle. By teaching middle-class women how to use the tools of coquetry, the Grand Coquette encouraged them to imagine a new relationship between respectability and sexuality.

The women's periodical introduced the Grand Coquette to the middle class. As part of a national press boom, the number of long-running women's and fashion magazines quadrupled between 1890 and 1914.[21] Journals varied widely in coverage, scope, and price; however, most featured aspirational models of womanhood. Luxury publications like *Femina* enticed the worldly reader with elaborate illustrations, early photojournalism, and high-society reportage. At four francs per issue, *Femina* cost at least twice as much as most women's magazines.[22] Meanwhile, less ostentatious, more modestly priced (ranging from 1 to 2 francs per issue) journals like the weekly *La mode pratique* (1891–1939) and the bimonthly *Chiffons* (1907–1932) also flourished, reaching forty-two thousand and two hundred thousand readers, respectively.[23] Both types of magazines cultivated a broad middle-class readership; however, it was the glamorous society magazine *Femina* that most elaborately promoted the Grand Coquette as an enviable model of respectable womanhood.

Founded in 1901, *Femina* quickly established itself as one of the most popular bimonthly women's reads. The journal provided a fascinating collage of French society and featured articles by some of the era's most revered writers and personalities. Additionally, *Femina* positioned the Grand Coquette alongside female telephone operators, postal workers, dentists, manicurists, actresses, and *midinettes,* and it presented her as the fashionable "girl of today" in an effort to make her culturally relevant to middle-class readers. In a series of articles devoted to her in the first decade of the twentieth century, contributors—including Gyp, Victor Margueritte, and Colette Yver—correlated the coquette with the "ideal" French girl and compared this "young woman of tomorrow" with both her antecedents and her American counterpart. Madeleine, a frequent *Femina* contributor, explained that "under the influence of modern life," of "cosmopolitanism" and "Americanism," a new, less fragile French girl had emerged. Unlike the "plastic," "sporty," and seemingly generic American, "Miss Fluffy Ruffles," the French girl possessed a strong "vie intérieure," a "grace," "simplicity," and "morality" that revealed itself in her modest smile.[24]

Yet the extravagant beauties who, by gracing the pages of women's magazines, gave life to this image—la belle Otero, Liane de Pougy, and Cécile Sorel, for example—were anything but modest. Perhaps no one better embodied the Grand Coquette than the celebrated actress Cécile Sorel, who adeptly played the character onstage and off. In 1908, Sorel's suggestively sinewy, full-body silhouette appeared alongside the text for a *Femina* article entitled "Les grandes coquettes." In it, she explained that playing the coquette onstage was one of the actress's most challenging roles. Not only did the Grand Coquette possess certain physical qualities—clear complexion, lustrous hair, and well-defined features—but she also had an audacity, a special charm that could be difficult to portray. For playwrights, the Grand Coquette was an emotionally complex woman who "wants to be loved, but she does not like it [the need/desire to be loved]."[25]

Yet even celebrated coquettes like Sorel had detractors. The spunky blonde, renowned for overplaying her lines and inflating her importance, found herself the object of ridicule in 1921 when a famous caricaturist chose her as his subject. The *Pittsburgh Post-Gazette* reported that upon seeing her image displayed at the *Comic Artists' Exhibition*, the insulted actress attempted to smash it with a jeweled bon-bon box. Upset by her exaggerated features and elongated face, she told reporters: "This caricature is an offense against beauty, which is the most precious possession in France. It was my duty to show my resentment against it, not only on my own account but as a representation of womanhood, of elegance and beauty."[26] The reporter added insult to injury by questioning whether Sorel's reputation was deserved in the first place. "She is a woman of remarkable distinction, grace, and elegance," the writer began. "France generally regards her as a true beauty, although critical persons might object to accepting this statement without qualification. Mademoiselle has an aggressively aquiline nose on her charming face, her chin is noticeable sharp, and her eyelids have a droop that is distinguished rather than beautiful."[27] These critiques notwithstanding, for decades Sorel provided a model of feminine beauty that men admired and that women sought to emulate.

Although they may never approach Sorel's prestige, middle-class women nevertheless hoped that they could, through diligent grooming and fashionable dress, successfully transform themselves into coquettes. To help them achieve this aim, *Femina* included features devoted to all sorts of beauty practices. In 1902, Maurice Ravidat told readers what to expect in "Chez la manicure." Ravidat assured readers that it was "a legitimate feminine coquetry to have beautiful hands."[28] To illustrate this point, he interviewed a manicurist and provided a step-by-step explanation for how to properly care for one's hands and nails. In March 1903, another contributor explored "l'art du maquillage." This unattributed writer chronicled how the actress transformed herself into "la grande coquette." Although she included nine photos of the Grand Coquette and devoted two full pages to the transformation process, the journalist reminded readers in her last paragraph that makeup appropriate for the stage would be "disastrous for a day on the boulevard."[29] Articles also often explained that cosmetics were instrumental for concealing an aging body. In "Quelques préceptes de beauté," for example, Smilis explained how new procedures in massage therapy could alleviate signs of aging. Perpetuating beauty ideals, introducing readers to new practices, and recommending products, *Femina* exposed the constant work required to create the Grand Coquette.

To carry out this work, readers could rely on one of the many beauty aids, systems, or institutes advertised in the magazine. Among the numerous product advertisements, women could erase wrinkles with A. Autard creams, mask imperfections with La Diaphane and Neige de Noël rice powders, whiten smiles with Odol or Gibbs tooth elixirs, or manage hair with Pétrole Hahn. Ads commonly featured beauty regimes as well as products. For example, in 1910, the "famous beauty specialist" Harriet Meta Smith provided *Femina* subscribers a coupon for her "complete information" guide for making "wrinkles disappear." This exclusive, free offer was promoted in the ad through testimonials from the Comtesse de Kergommeaux of Paris and Mme. Lluvia of Spain and through mention of awards received from various Universal Exposition juries.[30] If products and regimes failed to produce the desired effects, women could rely on one of Paris's new beauty institutes. Ads for Madame Adair's institute could be found in almost every issue of *Femina* in the first decade of the twentieth century. These were soon accompanied by solicitations for the institutes of Helena Rubinstein and Lina Cavalieri.

Features devoted to actresses, models, socialites, and even courtesans were commonplace in many women's magazines, and, like them, *Femina* provided a special lens into France's emerging celebrity culture. Responding to public interest in fashion and fashionable people, the press launched a "star system" that centered on Parisian elites. "The society columns of *Le Journal* and the *Figaro,* and many kindred publications," the culture and fashion critic Octave Uzanne explained, "huddle together the most illustrious princesses, the best-known courtesans, the most fashionable actresses, and the most retiring ladies of the wealthy bourgeoisie, in a most . . . easy-going fashion."[31] By elevating fashionable women to the level of princesses and the *grand bourgeoisie,* the press welcomed transgressive actresses and seamy courtesans into polite society.[32] As ladies of fashion, the Grand Coquettes were idolized as unique specimens of the feminine; however, as morally suspect entertainers, they retained their status as social pariahs. Caught between two worlds, the Grand Coquette revealed the growing pains of a French beauty culture that simultaneously promoted female pleasure and desire while insisting that those pleasures and desires remain locked within the bounds of middle-class conventions.

This contradiction was nothing new for actresses who had long held a complicated relationship to polite society. In the eighteenth century, the actress epitomized chic at the same time that she signaled sexual availability and moral depravity. For much of the nineteenth century, she was constructed as a dangerous, erotic figure. This characterization was due in part to her frequent forays into prostitution (recall Nana) but also to her ability to please men—her coquettishness. The actress's visibility increased in the 1850s, when technological developments in lithography and photography made reproducing her image less expensive. Consumers found these photos available for purchase in the photography shops and store windows of the *grandes boulevards*. These images connected the actress even more concretely to the commercial marketplace and transformed her into a commodity offstage as well as on. Under the Second Empire, a regime whose focus on public spectacle, grandeur, and national prosperity mimicked the actress's libertine heritage, the performer's sexualized body, in print and in person, attracted patrons and sold theater tickets.[33]

It was during the late nineteenth century, however, when theatergoing established itself as one of the most popular forms of entertainment for men *and* women, that the social standing of the actress was raised to that of her status as sex symbol. Indeed, between 1880 and 1910, an average of five hundred thousand people went to Parisian theaters every week, and during this same period, 274 café concerts operated in the city.[34] Female theatergoers shopped in the city's department stores, frequented hair salons, dabbled in cosmetics, admired stage fashions, and increasingly asked to know more about the styles and the women who wore them. Journalists quickly responded to the demand for this information and, by filling magazines with images of actresses, inadvertently strengthened commercial ties between the world of fashion and the world of theater.

Nonetheless, journalists, who themselves fought to be taken seriously, faced a dilemma when reporting on women of the theater. How could they disclose the seedy private lives of actresses to bourgeois readers without either condoning their "unwomanly" behaviors or jeopardizing the careers of both the actress and themselves? In the end, journalists portrayed actresses as "intimate strangers." They focused on the everyday domestic lives of these women rather than on their experiences in the theater or in the boudoir. By crafting stories about the actress as an ordinary, respectable woman, journalists created common ground between her and bourgeois readers. Yet, they tempered this depiction with descriptions of the celebrity's attractiveness and exceptional professional skill so that the bourgeois woman could not identify too closely with her idol. The press thus produced the Grand Coquette by choreographing the actress's imagined reality. On the one hand, it cloaked her experiences in the illusion of ordinariness while sweeping away transgressions; on the other, it celebrated her exceptional talent and beauty to reinforce her larger-than-life stage persona. The net effect was that a middle-class woman could simultaneously identify with and disassociate from the Grand Coquette—she could emulate that which she admired and eschew that which she disdained.

The Grand Coquette was also featured in a new form of cultural entertainment—the periodical beauty contest. Early on, these contests drew participants exclusively from the pool of Parisian celebrities revered for their attractiveness. In 1896, for example, the lavish middle-class journal *Illustration* selected the most beautiful woman from among popular stage performers. Contestants were judged based on particular features (hair, complexion, body shape) as well as their overall "look." The winner was the teenaged starlet Cléo de Mérode, who beat out Sarah Bernhardt, la belle Otéro, and Réjane for the top honor. Mérode was selected because she symbolized not only a woman of the world, but one still innocent. Celebrated for this virtue, she offered a safe alternative to her more mature, presumably sexually experienced competitors.[35]

Following the success of contests like the one sponsored by *Illustration,* women's periodicals soon sponsored contests that featured ordinary women. In 1904, *Femina* reported on American beauty competitions, and three years later, in September 1907, the journal participated in an international contest launched by the *Chicago Tribune. Femina*'s contest for the most beautiful woman in France explicitly excluded "les beautés professionnelles," thus limiting the competition to amateurs. *Femina* required that a parent or a friend, rather than the participant herself, submit a recent photograph. An illustrious jury of journalists, photographers, and other beauty experts used these photos to determine the top contestants, who would be featured in the journal and awarded prizes.[36] Periodical contests were a relatively novel practice at this time; however, their popularity grew in the prewar years as ordinary women parlayed their pleasing profiles, hoping to appear in magazines alongside their idols.[37]

Yet not all periodicals portrayed the Grand Coquette in a positive light; several exposed her artificial and commercial character by comparing her to *la poupée*—a doll. In 1901, *La vie parisienne* devoted six two-page tracts to the "divine poupée" and mockingly chronicled a female's life as one that revolved around beautification and an endless quest to make herself into a doll.[38] Similarly, the January 10, 1902, cover of the satirical journal *Le charivari* featured three fashionable ladies looking through a toy-store window at a display of fashion dolls, *poupées à la mode* (the best-selling French toy of 1901).[39] Two of the women appear immersed in the display, while a third coyly stares out at the reader, supporting the caption, "It is we who are the most beautiful dolls!" An eroticized image of woman, conspicuous by her elaborate dress, worldly expression, and completely visible makeup, the inanimate *poupée à la mode* replicated the real-life Grand Coquette. By conflating the Grand Coquette with this doll, the *Charivari* caricaturist revealed a conservative backlash toward the liberated woman.

As the *Charivari* comparison illustrates, the pleasure-seeking coquette inspired debates about woman's role in both the sexual and commercial economy. Vilified as a hypersexual narcissist who mercilessly teased and indiscriminately seduced, the coquette was envisioned as a dangerous social pariah. Why, then, would the Grand Coquette come to represent a desirable model of womanhood at the turn of the century? To answer this question necessitates understanding how commercial beauty culture produced the Grand Coquette as a mass spectacle. Through the dual process of spectacularization and commodification—making the coquette legible in text and image and constructing her as an object to be visually consumed—women's periodicals like *Femina* minimized her sexual and social threat by making her knowable. Featuring the Grand Coquette alongside advice columns related to self-care and product advertisements for cleansers, concealers, and cosmetics, magazines exposed the tools in the coquette's arsenal, in much the same way that Zola and Manet exposed Venus's. In so doing, they demystified the coquette and revealed coquetry as a learned practice.

Coquetry as practice, as a form of respectable beauty work, thus demonstrated how cosmetics made commodified beauty accessible and acceptable to all women. Magazines not only illuminated the practical work of coquetry; they also represented this work as a key element of woman's self-performance. Showing how the coquette created herself through intricately scripted, highly stylized rituals and behaviors, magazines acknowledged her exceptional beauty at the same time that they used it to domesticate her pursuit of pleasure. Thus produced, the Grand Coquette offered an exciting, if somewhat tamer model of womanhood than the Nineteenth-Century Venus.

She showed ordinary women how, through reconciling coquetry with morality, they could "keep the hearts" that they "had conquered."

THE BEAUTY COUNTESS

Produced in the high arts, literature, and the press, the Nineteenth-Century Venus and the Grand Coquette proffered reproducible models of womanhood; however, they provided only limited instruction as to how middle-class women could achieve such transformations. By contrast, self-proclaimed Beauty Countesses authored modestly priced, meticulously detailed breviaries and manuals that taught women how to make themselves beautiful. Posing as aristocrats, Beauty Countesses played upon established associations between beauty and luxury to peddle their advice books and pamphlets to eager middle-class consumers. At the same time, by emphasizing values of work and hygiene, they converted cosmetics from symbols of aristocratic excess into tools of bourgeois industry. Thus blurring class distinctions, Beauty Countesses transformed woman's pursuit of beauty from a frivolous self-indulgence into a necessary and respectable female labor.

Beauty Countesses authored dozens of popular beauty books at the turn of the twentieth century. At the helm of this explosion, the Comtesse de Norville, the Comtesse de Tramar, the Comtesse de Gencé, the Baronne Staffe, and the Vicomtesse Nacla penned numerous manuals that went through several editions and printings.[40] Yet these Beauty Countesses had little real connection to the aristocracy. Among the aforementioned authors, only the Comtesse de Tramar (Marie Fanny de Lamarque de Lagarrigue baronne d'Ysarn de Capdeville marquise de Villefort) was a certifiable French noblewoman. Although the true identities of the Comtesse de Norville and the Vicomtesse de Nacla are uncertain, the modest origins of the Comtesse de Gencé (Marie Louise Pouyollon) and of the Baronne Staffe (Blanche Soyer) are well documented. Whether these writers were genuine nobles is ultimately less important than how, by posing as such, they used these titles to signal social authority. These authors were not only advisors who held the attention of thousands of readers, but also performers who constructed identities not as baronesses or vicomtesses in the original sense, but as Beauty Countesses—the most elite, the most glamorous, of all self-care experts.

Beauty Countesses targeted a middle-class audience and in so doing found themselves competing with health-care professionals for readers. Rather than rely on scientific expertise or professional training as their male counterparts had done, Beauty Countesses drew on their experiences as women to claim authority. Nevertheless, Beauty Countesses appealed to readers by emphasizing the merits of personal cleanliness and by including chapters in their manuals devoted to bathing, shampooing, oral hygiene, and pore respiration. They, too, encouraged the use of natural products, filled their manuals with recipes, and provided lengthy expositions on the aesthetics of feminine beauty. Additionally, they introduced women to new products, encouraged them to experiment with innovative techniques and services, and taught them, in step-by-step fashion, how to carry out hygienic beauty regimes. Although they might echo health-care professionals, Beauty Countesses nevertheless spoke in a univocal, female voice.

Beauty Countesses regarded self-care as a social imperative. In *Le bréviaire de la femme: Pratiques secrets de la beauté* (1903), the Comtesse de Tramar explained that the pretty girl was "indispensible to society." It was, moreover, her "social role" to prevent wrinkles, avoid fluctuations of body weight, and maintain hygiene.[41] The Comtesse de Norville extended the notion of feminine beauty as social obligation by linking it to familial duty, religious sentiment, and medical prescription. She opened *Les coulisses de la beauté: Comment la femme séduit* (in its third edition in 1895) with the assertion that a young woman's beauty was "the pride" of a nice family. Once a woman reached adulthood, she added, her husband and children would "desire it." Cultivating her beauty was not only in the interest of her family; it also embodied the "symbolic forms" put forth in religion and complied with the standards of good health.

Beauty Countesses brought respectability to artifice and self-care, not by merely evoking its social benefits but also by explicitly promoting it as a female pleasure. Beauty Countesses armed woman with recipes, products, and techniques that enabled her to fully realize her inner coquette. Specifically, by connecting *plaisir* (pleasure) and *devoir* (duty), they played on bourgeois notions of industry to legitimize woman's use of artifice and to transform coquetry into a respectable feminine practice. As the Comtesse de Gencé so eloquently elucidated: "An honest woman has the right to be a coquette, because coquetry as understood today, isn't contradictory to morality, good sense, or taste. . . . In a sense, to be a coquette is next to being well-bred."[42] By linking coquetry to honesty and good breeding, countesses moved far beyond the sanitized language of hygiene and cleanliness favored by health-care professionals to explicitly correlate feminine beauty with sexuality and even female desire.

Beauty Countesses borrowed liberally from a cultural cosmology that portrayed the pursuit of beauty as fundamental to woman's nature. In *Brevet de femme chic* (1907), Baronne Staffe maintained that the "chic woman wants to please" because it is "in her nature" to do so.[43] Likewise, Norville argued that the "desire to be beautiful was innate within women."[44] She supported the adages that "physical beauty reflects a beautiful soul" and that the "face reflects the thoughts, character, and heart of the individual."[45] Beauty was more than a reflection of a woman's character; it was, according to Staffe, her responsibility. She reminded readers that "you have a mission to please and to charm." "You," she continued, "are ideal in the rude life of man; do not fall from the pedestal upon which he has placed you."[46] In these lamentations, Beauty Countesses reinforced the notion that the pursuit of beauty was fundamental to woman's nature—in short, it was part of her sex.

Indeed, Beauty Countesses deemed beauty work important because only a clean and healthy female body would attract desirable sexual partners. In *A la conquête du bonheur!* (1912), Tramar instructed women in "la coquetterie utilitaire" because, as she explained, "women always tied notions of romantic love to beauty of appearance" and so "coquetry [became] the indispensable auxiliary of beauty."[47] She compared the use of artifice to a "sport that requires finesse" and a "complex science" before arguing frankly that the attractive woman need "accept the advantages and obligations of her social role by conserving her beauty and upholding the illusion for all of her admirers."[48] Moreover, once she attracted a partner, he should find her always "fresh and beautiful," "pleasing," "charm[ing]," and "virtu[ous]."[49] The key to "conjugal happiness," coquetry, according to the Vicomtesse Nacla, should be the "primary task of the spouse."[50]

Beauty Countesses also charged women with teaching their husbands and children hygienic practices and values. Madame Boeswilwald acknowledged this imperative when she instructed readers in how to bathe themselves and their offspring, cautioning them not to wash with their children for fear of transmitting germs.[51] Like washing, beauty habits were also to be passed from mother to child. The appearance of a young girl, Boeswilwald explained, depended on her mother because "beauty care began at the moment of birth."[52]

Tramar maintained that it was every mother's job to "attach an extreme importance to hygienic care" because it was through these labors that women could combat childhood ailments and contagious diseases.[53] In *La femme dans la famille* (1900), Baronne Staffe urged women to always listen to mother's advice.[54] Charging women with the corporeal care of husbands and offspring, Beauty Countesses reiterated the notion that beauty work served the middle-class family.

Although they acknowledged the diligent work required to make women beautiful, Beauty Countesses celebrated beautification as a personal indulgence. Certainly, women wanted to attract male admirers and please their husbands; however, as Tramar pointed out in *Que veut la femme? Être jolie, être aimée et dominer* (1911), women also regarded their physical appearance as "the exterioration of the *moi intime.*" At first blush, Tramar's claim appears to merely reiterate Romantic and even religious notions of beauty that equated a virtuous soul with a pleasing face. Yet in the context of a manual that brazenly foregrounds "what a woman wants," Tramar's association between body and self must be more carefully considered. Tramar believed that woman hid her "intimate sensations" (her thoughts, emotions, and personal desires) behind a "deliberate mask" that, when it "functioned automatically," could "master nature."[55] Tending the body, maintaining the mask to protect a vulnerable *moi intime,* was for Tramar an empowering act. Through the practice of the toilette, woman cultivated a special relationship between an interior self and an exterior body; this relationship not only permitted woman to "be liked by and to dominate" the opposite sex but also opened a space for developing woman's sexual power.

Tramar's evocations found particular resonance in a culture inundated with images of nude women. Impressionist art, the growth of photography, the proliferation of actress profiles on boulevard broadsides and life-size posters, and the wide-scale circulation of pornography had the French looking at unclothed female bodies like never before. Not only were nudes, like those shown in *Olympia* and *Nana,* becoming commonplace in the media and in public, they were also becoming more visible in the privacy of the middle-class home. By the end of the nineteenth century, the full-length mirror (*l'amoire à glace*) became a fixture in the boudoirs of respectable households. For the first time, a modest young woman could observe her entire nude body—she could, quite literally, finally see all of herself. A consequence of this activity, as Diane Barthel has so eloquently explained, is that the mirror came to symbolize the feminine. A necessity rather than a vanity, "the mirror reflected the commandment that women see themselves as others see them" and rendered women simultaneously critics and objects.[56] Remarkably, as the toilette became an increasingly private, hidden affair, one of its most important instruments, the looking glass, made the nude female body more visible than ever before.

Rather than retreat from discoveries made in front of the mirror, Beauty Countesses encouraged women to address them head-on and to even luxuriate in their revelations. Gencé believed that for a woman to create her "personal illusion," she needed to use the *cabinet de toilette* as a place "to fantasize and escape into luxury, to bask in the eternal feminine."[57] She considered the sacred space of the beauty cabinet not only an "artist's loge where no one else should enter" but also as "a confessional" where women encountered their true selves, flaws and all.[58] The magic of the toilette and of the space where it was performed—the "place of silence and mystery" to Nacla, the "mysterious temple" to Tramar—tied woman into the mystical and portrayed the pursuit of personal beauty as a spiritual journey.[59] Through analogies like these, Beauty Countesses envisioned beautification as nothing less than an awakening of the female self.

The beauty cabinet may have been imagined as a numinous world and the products within it as magical potions capable of transforming ordinary women into goddesses, but in reality, the Beauty Countesses understood that "to be beautiful is always work."[60] Gencé advised that beauty cabinets were to be "clean and microbe-free," while "products should be stored in crystal containers" and "arranged properly."[61] The cabinet, Tramar added, should be filled with the appropriate products—almond pastes, cucumber pomades, toothpastes, and cleansing powders.[62] "Given the innumerable beauty products available," Tramar explained, "it is important that each woman choose her products judiciously."[63] The toilette itself should require the better part of a morning, and it should be conducted "tastefully and orderly in a rational manner."[64]

The diligent bourgeois should also minister to the body in a careful and systematic manner. Tramar urged woman to "study her physique" and to view her body as a machine and herself as the mechanic charged with keeping it running.[65] Bodily care required such effort because "few women are born beautiful," and it is she who "creates the best mirage [who] is prettiest."[66] To help women achieve the "best mirage," Beauty Countesses filled their lengthy manuals (they ranged from two hundred to six hundred pages) with detailed regimes. Gencé, for example, proposed nine steps for conducting the toilette in a rational manner: (1) Bathe; (2) frictions and massage; (3) wash hands; (4) wash legs and feet; (5) clean mouth, throat, and teeth; (6) clean neck, shoulders, and arms; (7) face, eyes, ears; (8) hair; and (9) hands and nails.[67] If Gencé's program was extensive, then Boeswilwald's was exhaustive. Her nightly regime alone included an astounding twenty-one steps![68] While not all guides were so rigid in their direction, almost all of them were divided into sections or chapters devoted to specific areas of the body. Writers delegated from two to fifty pages per body part, allotting, for instance, ten pages for hair care and another forty for dental hygiene. Through these intricate regimes, Beauty Countesses provided women with a comprehensive guide to self-care at the same time that they fragmented the female body. By attending to each individual fragment, the industrious middle-class woman could create a harmonious, cohesive whole.

In their prescriptive guides, Beauty Countesses helped establish the boundaries of respectable womanhood by presenting beauty as *devoir* (duty)—an acceptable form of middle-class woman's work. Beauty Countesses equated beauty with the eternal feminine, and they elevated it to the natural and to the divine. However, as manual authors, these women brokered in the contingent, in the mutable, and they acknowledged that woman was not born beautiful but rather became so if provided the right environment, tools, and training. By affording such careful attention to the spaces, products, and rituals of beautification, Beauty Countesses reinforced the idea that, although she may enjoy it, keeping up appearances was ultimately a woman's work.

Importantly, Beauty Countesses garnered respectability for this feminine mission by posing as members of the social elite. The implication of this pose was twofold. By playing with appearances, Beauty Countesses claimed noble status to authenticate their advice. In demonstrating artifice's role in the creation and performance of new identities, Beauty Countesses pointed to both the liberating and constraining aspects of beauty play. On the one hand, beauty opened up possibilities for self-exploration; on the other, beauty's homogenized practices reinforced the long-held belief that beauty was the domain and the responsibility of every Frenchwoman. As the Comtesse de Tramar expressed it, with so many people to please and with so many ways to beautify, respectable French women "had no excuse for being ugly."[69]

The Work of Beauty

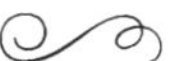

Through the related figures of the Nineteenth-Century Venus, the Grand Coquette, and the Beauty Countess, Manet and Zola, women's magazines, and beauty manuals articulated broader cultural concerns about middle-class womanhood. Located at the intersection of the sexual and commercial economies of late-nineteenth-century France, these models of womanhood exposed current anxieties regarding woman's sexual desire, public visibility, and self-indulgence. The Nineteenth-Century Venus coupled woman's pursuit of pleasure with the acquisition of sexual power. In full command of the viewer, in control of her body, and mistress of her boudoir, Olympia asserted her sexual agency. In transformation, Nana showed women how to create themselves as objects and subjects of carnal desire, while in her autoerotic performance she demonstrated how to find sexual gratification in the absence of men. By making a spectacle of her body and encouraging ordinary women to do the same, the Grand Coquette blurred arbitrary boundaries between public and private. On the public stage, these women entered popular consciousness, while through the mass-circulated magazine, they entered the bourgeois home, offering up infinite images of corporeal beauty for respectable women to admire. Finally, the Beauty Countess taught women that the same beauty work intended to benefit class and family could also please woman herself. Bridging the gulf between reality and fantasy, Beauty Countesses showed women how to achieve their own beauty ideals.

Through the work of beauty, the Nineteenth-Century Venus, the Grand Coquette, and the Beauty Countess more than pushed the boundaries of social probity, however; they unapologetically challenged the middle-class status quo. At first blush, the sexually charged Nineteenth-Century Venus appeared as the antithesis to the respectable woman, even though both represented submissive objects of male desire. Yet, working-class prostitutes like Olympia and Nana called into question the notion that women could be naturally devoid of sexual feeling. In so doing, the Nineteenth-Century Venus opened a space where even respectable women could contemplate sexual agency—for by playing her prescribed social role, the dutiful wife determined which expectations and behaviors would be permissible in the conjugal bedroom. In short, she might establish the rules for "keeping the heart" that she "had conquered."

Whereas the Nineteenth-Century Venus resided simultaneously in the high arts and in popular culture, the Grand Coquette and the Beauty Countess were more firmly positioned inside France's commercial beauty culture. As creators, products, and consumers of this culture, the Grand Coquette and the Beauty Countess manipulated its tools and strategies to demand visibility and to legitimize their pursuit of pleasure. Active and public, invested in both consumer society as well as in her own commodification, the Grand Coquette proposed a model of womanhood diametrically opposed to the passive, sheltered, middle-class wife. The Grand Coquette's glamour, beauty, and notoriety, however, appealed precisely to the reputable lady who, through her own social invisibility, suffered the tedium of quotidian domesticity. Thus the Grand Coquette, as a female fantasy of the feminine, encouraged women to look beyond the banal and to envision (even if only imaginary) new identities. The Beauty Countess echoed this call and showed women how they could, in reality, create new selves through a commitment to beauty work. They suggested that all women possessed correctable corporeal imperfections, and they offered readers practical advice for surmounting these deficiencies. Celebrating the tools of commercial beauty culture, the Grand Coquette and the Beauty Countess taught ordinary women that beauty was not a biological blessing but an achievable goal.

Ultimately, the work of beauty expanded the range of acceptable social roles available to women by disseminating competing discourses of femininity that, in a subtle and sophisticated way, subverted the prevailing gender ideology. By evoking the truly exceptional—the prostitute, the coquette, the aspiring socialite—as viable models of womanhood, the sources above both acknowledged and legitimized feminine desire. Rather than deny woman's capacity for pleasure, moreover, these media endeavored to domesticate it—to overcome the obstacles of sexuality, visibility, and self-indulgence not through eradication but through rearticulation. Destabilizing the social order from within, this strategic move resulted in no less than a paradigm shift in which beauty functioned not as a marker of woman's subordination but as a route to social legibility and sexual power. The celebrated author and self-proclaimed beauty expert Sidonie-Gabrielle Colette called upon similar strategies and used her own exceptional relationship to beauty to illustrate how women could create themselves as both independent women and autonomous individuals in the early twentieth century. How Colette engaged both beauty work and the work of beauty will be the focus of part II.

PART II

Exceptional Beauty

> Nowhere else in the world, Claudine, are women as pretty as they are in Paris! (Let's leave Montigny out of it, darling . . .) It's in Paris that you see the most fascinating faces whose beauty is waning—women of forty, frantically made-up and tight-laced, who have kept their delicate noses and eyes like a young girl's. Women who let themselves be stared at with a mixture of pleasure and bitterness.
>
> —Colette, *Claudine Married*

In the above passage from Colette's popular and scandalous Claudine series, Rezi, the protagonist's friend and soon-to-be lover, ebulliently associates beauty with the aging female body.[1] Only in Paris, she contends, do women's bodies so honestly and vividly reveal the eternal contest between youth—signified in "delicate noses" and "eyes like a young girl's"—and maturity, concealed partially behind "frantically made-up" faces. The "fascinating faces" of these "women of forty" enchant Rezi not only because they evoke a "beauty [that] is waning," but also because they occupy a privileged place in the specular economy of the modern city. These are faces made intentionally for display, bodies fashioned deliberately to absorb the ubiquitous, anonymous gaze that permeates the bustling metropolis. Positioned firmly between adolescence and old age, moreover, these women are so fully cognizant of the limits of their corporeal advantages that, though complicit in the performance, they exhibit their faces and bodies with a "mixture of pleasure and bitterness." And so it is through the passing comment of this relatively minor character that Colette eloquently articulates what would become a central theme of her later literary work as well as a lifelong personal quest: reconciling pleasure with bitterness and youth with maturity to create oneself as both a woman and an individual.[2]

In her endeavor to author narratives of independent womanhood, Colette encountered formidable cultural impediments. Foremost among these obstacles was a pervasive and entrenched nineteenth-century liberal ideology of womanhood that codified woman's subordination.[3] Premised on a binary classification of sexual difference, this inflexible ideology evoked biology to legitimize complementary social roles for middle-class women and men. In so doing, it became the basis for woman's exclusion from politics and much of public life, and it undermined the notion that women could exist independently from men. Indeed, a significant corollary to this ideology was the assertion that women be self*less,* meaning not only that they devote themselves entirely to family, home, and nation but also that they renounce the possibility of cultivating a female self altogether.

By the time Colette began writing novels in the 1890s, critiques of this ideology, and of woman's role in society more generally, had emerged from a variety of sources. Feminists and social reformers disputed women's limited participation in politics; doctors and hygienists acknowledged women's importance to the health and welfare of the nation; and the feminine press and various commercial and business interests encouraged women's economic agency. One of the more creative and insidious challenges to arise, however, materialized in the figure of the New Woman.[4] Caricatured in periodicals and featured in popular novels and plays, the New Woman was a cultural icon, perhaps even more alive in the European imaginary than on the boulevards of its major cities.[5] As a vibrant and blossoming genre, New Woman literature promised fresh female life plots, exhilarating ways of living in the world, and exciting alternatives to domesticity. Too frequently, however, these promises went unrealized as authors simply imitated Henrik Ibsen's model in *A Doll's House* (1878), in which the New Woman's story ends at the moment that she exits the conjugal home. Thus, even in fiction, imagining a woman's postdomestic life proved difficult.[6]

More than a rhetorical device or allegorical symbol, however, new women were also a social reality. Indeed, scholars have demonstrated the indivisible bond between the embodied new woman and her cultural (New Woman) image. Women who were considered "new," either in the media or on the boulevard, shared a set of characteristics that marked them as exceptional. Whether real or imagined, the New Woman was, as Mary Louise Roberts lucidly explains, the "primarily urban, middle-class French woman" who fell under public scrutiny in the 1890s and early 1900s. Although sometimes set apart by marital status, profession, or political inclination, "all of these women challenged the regulatory norms of gender by living unconventional lives and by doing work outside the home that was coded masculine in French culture."[7]

By these criteria, Colette was both a new woman and an author of New Woman literature. She understood that woman's struggle to achieve autonomy would remain unrealized until her story was no longer tethered to the hermeneutic yoke of domesticity. Colette promoted woman's self-fulfillment and self-development; and she popularized a performative notion of identity that challenged an ethos in which biology was destiny and the self was an essentialized certainty rather than a dynamic potentiality. Unlike many writers of New Woman literature, however, Colette did not conclude her stories at the moment of departure from the bourgeois home. In her fiction, Colette eschewed the middle-class household entirely. Choosing rather to explore the liminal recesses of society—its theaters, boulevards, and brothels—Colette depicted worlds that decentered the middle-class home (and, by extension, the gender norms that regulated it). By rendering the domestic peripheral in her writing, Colette effectively destabilized the master narrative of liberal gender ideology and opened a conceptual space for envisioning new models of French womanhood.

Colette imagined the New Woman's complex relationship to society as an arduous contest between the dictated norms of gender and a feminine self in which subjectivity emerged independently of culturally constructed paradigms. To discover how to become a self *and* a woman, Colette suggests, one must shed the status of "other" entirely; she must assert personal sovereignty and reclaim the very idea of the feminine. For Colette, returning the feminine to a position of authority required a new conceptual framework, a new lexicon of selfhood in which beauty and womanhood could be harmoniously reconciled. Assuming that the autonomous female self could only be accessed once the social conventions regulating feminine beauty were amended, Colette, in both her life and her work, relentlessly scrutinized the politics of feminine self-production.

Part II examines how Colette, as a writer, performer, and cosmetics entrepreneur, equated beauty work with the work of being a woman. Providing a close textual analysis of *La vagabonde* (1910) and *Chéri* (1920), chapter 3 analyzes how, through her tormented protagonists Renée and Léa, Colette evoked the aging female body as a critical site for understanding the symbiotic relationship between beauty and power. On the one hand, beauty empowers Colette's heroines, enabling them to defy convention, to earn a living (in the music hall and the boudoir, respectively), and to pursue personal pleasures. On the other, beauty (and, more to the point, its loss) precipitates a profound crisis of identity for women who too readily associate good looks and well-made bodies with an authentic self. By examining the relationship between power and beauty as a problem of new womanhood, Colette's novels highlight how contemporary notions of aging paradoxically enabled and impeded woman's self-production.

Whereas, in chapter 3, the aging female body elucidates the contest between beauty and power, in chapter 4, woman's everyday encounters with makeup illustrate the extent to which appearance and selfhood became indivisible in the female imaginary. Exploring some of Colette's lesser-studied writings—her music-hall short stories, her *fait divers* publications in the French press, and her personal impressions about and publicity for her beauty business, I investigate how Colette mobilized cosmetics to illuminate the arduous labors through which women, from the most exceptional actress to the most humble housewife, struggle to produce female selves.

In each of these endeavors, Colette offers a unique lens for understanding the relationship between women and commercial beauty culture in the early twentieth century. Although beauty work figured prominently in the daily lives of many middle-class women, very few of them actually wrote about it. Colette's novels, short stories, and press articles, therefore, open a window onto woman's personal engagement with beauty work that would otherwise remain closed. Moreover, whereas Colette's characters, in their softly uttered asides and unspoken anxieties, reveal the intimate, her focus on music-hall performers and courtesans highlights intersections between beauty and commerce that came to define celebrity. Finally, as the proprietor of her own beauty institute and manufacturer of her own cosmetics line, Colette revealed beauty's centrality to the ordinary business of becoming "nothing but a woman."

3

Colette and the Contradictions of "Well-Made" Bodies

Two more hours of beauty in front of you—
don't you think that's worth having?
—Colette, *L'entrave*

In *Mes apprentissages* (1936), Colette confided that "occasionally, in my extreme youth, I found myself sighing to 'be somebody.' If I had had the courage to express my wish fully, I should have said 'somebody else.' But I soon gave it up. I have never succeeded in becoming somebody else."[1] Demonstrative of Colette's playfulness, her proclamation here is ostensibly more misleading than revealing. An esteemed member of the French literati, an acclaimed stage performer, and an internationally known celebrity, when she penned this confession at age sixty, Colette had indisputably established herself as "somebody." Despite her protestations to the contrary, moreover, she also managed, through her acting career but even more enduringly through her fiction, to continually reinvent herself as "somebody else."

Acknowledging the semiautobiographical character of Colette's fiction, scholars have reasoned that through the visceral act of writing—of literally and metaphorically producing textual somebodies—Colette created protagonists who mirrored her own anxieties. Anne Freadman's prudent caution against reading Colette's fiction uncritically *as* autobiography notwithstanding, many readers continue to search novels like *La vagabonde* (1910) and *Chéri* (1920) for evidence of Colette's "textual selfhood."[2] Certainly, Colette herself encouraged such elision; confessing that she drew upon her own life to create plots for her novels and admitting that "in them I call myself Renée Néré or else, prophetically, Léa."[3] As casually as Colette renders this admission, however, she denies that her novels reflect herself: "Does anyone imagine," she teases, ". . . that I am portraying myself?"[4]

Rather than provide an exhaustive account of Colette's literary oeuvre or detail the particulars of her fascinating life, this chapter examines two of her most complex and lauded protagonists, the formidable courtesan Léa de Lonval (*Chéri*) and the enigmatic actress Renée Néré (*La vagabonde*) to ascertain how Colette constructed the symbiotic relationship between beauty and power as a problem of new womanhood.[5] Marginalized by their professions and differentiated by their good looks and sexual availability, Léa and Renée used their "well-made bodies" to maneuver between classes, genders, and selves, and to live tenuously as autonomous individuals. Yet confronted with the loss of beauty that accompanies the advancement of age, Colette's heroines undergo agonizing metamorphoses.

Through Léa and Renée, Colette demonstrates that it is not the loss of beauty itself but rather woman's response to it that determines whether the aging body becomes an obstacle to feminine self-fulfillment or an opportunity for self-discovery. In desperation, both heroines initially turn to cosmetics to mask their imperfections. They learn, however, that while the superficial quick fix temporarily covers over physical blemishes, it does nothing to diminish the psychological scars accumulating beneath the skin's surface. Recognizing that artifice can neither resurrect their fading beauty nor rescue them from the inevitable progress of time, Léa and Renée have to come to terms with their aging female bodies.

This chapter examines how Colette evoked the contradictions of "well-made" bodies to author competing versions of womanhood. A seasoned courtesan who has spent a lifetime trading on her good looks, Léa reluctantly resigns herself to beauty's loss. Retiring from her profession rather than pursuing new ventures, Léa represents the woman for whom survival and the desire to live freely, on one's own terms, trumped all else. Renée, having come of age in the first decade of the twentieth century, relies as much on her craft, her *métier,* as upon her appearance to support herself.[6] Struggling not only to survive, but also to matter, Renée combats the challenges of aging by first becoming a self-sufficient vagabond and then succumbing to the shackle of love. Encapsulating Colette's own nostalgia for the past as well as her hope for the future, Léa and Renée defy convention at the same time that they reveal the tensions between woman's desire for independence and her desire to submit.

SUBVERSIVE BEAUTY: LÉA AND CHÉRI

Set amid the lavish parlors, trendy nightclubs, and fashionable resorts of prewar France, *Chéri* illuminates the decadent world of the Belle Époque courtesan. Although past their professional prime, the middle-aged prostitutes who serve as the main characters in the novel continue to enjoy lives of leisure and amusement. Financially secure and materially comfortable, Léa de Lonval and her set epitomize the power of beauty to free women from the strictures of social convention. Yet because these women derive professional value and personal worth exclusively from their appearance, a loss of beauty signals a considerable loss of power and provokes a full-blown identity crisis.

At first glance, *Chéri* merely documents the unraveling love affair between the forty-nine-year-old Léa de Lonval and her recently engaged twenty-four-year-old lover, Fred Peloux (a.k.a. Chéri). Closer scrutiny, however, reveals that it is not Chéri's pending nuptials, but the couple's inability to come to terms with Léa's aging body that has ended the six-year romance. Throughout their lives, beauty has marked Léa and Chéri as exceptional; it has provided them with a sense of self and place; and it has intimately linked them to one another. Idolized in her youth as a blonde goddess, Léa learned early how to use her "well-made body" to procure social status, to accumulate material wealth, and to pursue her personal pleasures.[7] The pampered son of another notorious courtesan (Léa's lifelong friend and rival Charlotte Peloux), Chéri, too, has used his beauty to live as he pleases. While Chéri has grown from adolescence into adulthood over the course of their relationship, however, Léa has constantly and vehemently battled the vagaries of middle age. Although still revered as an especially attractive *demimondaine,* Léa nevertheless confronts a thickening neck and a head of graying hair in the looking glass. In a relationship built on appearances, the potential loss of Léa's beauty is not only personally devastating; it also reveals a vulnerable seam in the lovers' sacred bond.

Opening the novel with an intimate interlude, Colette methodically details how physical beauty has united the couple. As the morning sun streams mercilessly into Léa's boudoir, Chéri prances around the room in his mistress's pearls. Chéri discovers himself "standing in front of a pier-glass framed in a space between two windows, gazing at the reflection of a very youthful, very good-looking young man" (91). Pleased with his reflection, he begins his disorderly toilette while Léa picks up "the fine pearls" with which Chéri had amused himself. Léa hopes that her young lover has not noticed "that her throat had thickened and was not nearly so white, with the muscles under the skin growing slack" (12). Unsettled by this admission, Léa calls herself a "market-gardener's wife" before considering "everything that she no longer loved in herself: the vivid complexion, healthy, a little too ruddy—an open-air complexion, well suited to emphasize the pure intensity of her eyes, with their varying shades of blue. Her proud nose still won her approval." Léa next inspects her mouth, "with its even row of teeth," and her "deep, confiding smile [that] one never tired of watching" before contemplating her "body, pink and white, endowed with the long legs and straight back of a naiad on an Italian fountain"; and "the dimpled hips, the high-slung breasts" that would last "till well after Chéri's wedding" (12–13).

Interrupted by Chéri's reentry into the bedroom, Léa quickly powders her face before turning her attention to finishing her lover's toilette. Treating him like a wayward schoolboy, Léa teases Chéri about his inability to effectively dress himself. She then takes over the project, noting that "[his] defenses were down. Blissful, languid, irresolute, supine, he surrendered again to a lazy happiness and closed his eyes." After arranging his tie, Léa "brushed the hair off his ears, combed a straighter parting in the bluish locks of his black hair, dubbed a little scent on his temples, and gave him a quick kiss" (15). Once she has sent Chéri on his way, Léa begins her own toilette, requesting the manicurist, enjoying a bath and a "spirit-rub scented with sandal-wood," and lingering over her Louis Seize looking glass (16). Although Léa would remark to her friends that "a well-made body lasts a long time," she could not prevent herself from anticipating, dreading, the moment when her "long time" would run out (13). Beneath the admiring gaze of her butler, she admits that he at least still finds her "beautiful." Despite this recognition, however, she indignantly claims: "No . . . No Longer. I have now to wear something white near my face, and very pale pink underclothes and tea-gowns. Beautiful! Pish . . . I hardly need to be that any longer" (17).

In this quietly murmured aside, Léa acknowledges the limits of a love affair based solely on beauty. Indeed, as Léa's meticulous attention to the couple's toilette, Chéri's inability to look away from his own exquisite reflection, and Léa's admiration of her lover's physique and her thorough scrutiny of her own confirm, the couple's relationship has hinged on producing and appreciating the beautiful body. Throughout the affair, Léa not only cultivated her own body but also transformed Chéri's weak adolescent frame into its current spectacular form. Léa has consistently plied Chéri with healthy foods and even hired him a personal trainer so that "the young body owed to her its renewed vigor" (35). In the early days of the romance, Léa had rejoiced "each morning his eyes and his mouth returned to life more beautiful, as though every waking, every embrace, had fashioned them anew! (36–37). As cultivator and disciplinarian of Chéri's body, Léa has exercised a mesmerizing power over her paramour. Under her guidance, the boy, physically and sexually, if not intellectually and emotionally, had grown into a man.

In reality, Chéri's subordination to Léa traps him in an interminable adolescence. Colette conveys the extent of Chéri's stunted development by attributing to him numerous conventionally feminine attributes. Obsessed with his own appearance, he revels in his status as pleasing decorative object. Given to tantrums that border on hysterics (that most prevalent female malady of the day), he resembles the spoiled child or the naïve young bride. Driven to excitement by luxuries and commodities (especially jewels and beauty products), he pleasures in adornment and frivolity. And, erratically fluctuating between submission and rebellion, he is impetuous, moody, and ruled entirely by emotion. Chéri's feminine qualities are counterbalanced by Léa's matronly ones: she dotes on him and encourages his insolence, she reins him in, she endures his excessive primping if only to complain about razor shavings in the sink, and, to shield him from the cruelties of the real world, she permits him to cling to the bosom of his "Nounoune" (10, 11).

Léa's influence over Chéri is threatened, however, by his pending marriage. Though Chéri barely acknowledges his fiancée and even expects to continue their affair, Léa fears that, older and sidelined, she will lose her relevance for him. Confounded by her thinly disguised anxiety, Chéri candidly reassures them both that she will "always be there . . . whenever I need you to do something for me." Predictably concerned with his own well-being, Chéri cannot imagine how or why his relationship with Léa should change. Léa does not dispel Chéri's belief that she will be available to him, but she makes it clear that she intends to carry on as usual and without him: "Do you expect me to go to Normandy and hide my grief? To pine away? To stop dying my hair?" (41).

Exploring the scandalous liaison between an aging prostitute and her young lover, Colette's novel brazenly transcended boundaries of social probity, subverting culturally embedded, class-based gender ideology to reconceptualize love, domesticity, and womanhood. Colette accomplishes this disruption by portraying Léa and Chéri's affair as perfectly normal even though it continuously complicates, rather than simply replicates, rules governing both conventional and transgressive heterosexual norms. Léa's uncontested power over Chéri paradoxically buttresses and inverts the typical courtesan/client paradigm. Controversial because it occurs outside of marriage, this type of relationship was nevertheless so common in Colette's Paris that it easily mirrored bourgeois conjugality. Admittedly more difficult to reproduce when a significant age difference existed between partners, as in the case of Léa and Chéri, this arrangement asserts itself as normative in Colette's novel nonetheless.

Conflating romantic love with maternal affection, moreover, Colette problematizes the affair by making it doubly subversive. As his lover, Léa helps bring Chéri into sexual maturity, but as a surrogate mother (ministering his toilette, reluctantly acknowledging his pending marriage, referring to Chéri boldly as the "son never born her"), she ultimately inhibits his ability to become a man. Empowering Léa within a relationship that is obviously extramarital and figuratively incestuous, Colette encourages a love and a model of womanly behavior that contemporaries would have considered indecent, even taboo. Here, then, beauty normalizes perversions, recasts relationships of power, and proposes new possibilities for women who do not desire to follow the dictates of domesticity. By normalizing the perverse, however, Léa and Chéri do not escape the domestic model inasmuch as they reproduce it in a different form. Beauty united the couple and cemented their subversive love, but it also cast the lovers as perfect complements.

COMPETITIVE BEAUTY: CHÉRI IN THE WORLD OF WOMEN

Colette further explores beauty's uncanny ability to simultaneously reinstate and upend norms by situating her drama in what appears to be a woman's world.[8] Set amid the commercial boudoirs, private parlors, and clandestine meeting places that comprised the courtesan's pleasure-filled underworld, the novel locates a peripheral reality (one that existed simultaneously beyond and within the bourgeois city) at the center of the narrative.[9] Colette's female characters, moreover, are "public women" in every sense. As career prostitutes, eager spectators, and literal streetwalkers, they belong to the urban landscape as much as it belongs to them. Free to move about the city in pursuit of their own amusements, these women enjoy physical mobility and social visibility. Indeed, the courtesan's relevance as well as her livelihood depended entirely on her ability to take advantage of these liberties. Yet geographic placement alone did not ensure that a woman would attract a suitor. Prostitutes had to stand out, to market themselves as alluring diversions within the city spectacle. Thus physical appearance became the authoritative measure of a courtesan's professional and personal worth. As Colette's courtesans attest, beauty and youth were more than mere aspirations for these women; they were tools of the trade, social and economic weapons, and potent symbols of selfhood.

In a pair of scenes that transpire in Charlotte Peloux's parlor, Colette deftly illustrates how, despite sharing a marginal social space and posing as amicable colleagues, courtesans regarded one another first and foremost as bitter rivals. The first scene, which depicts Charlotte and Marie-Laure's negotiation of Chéri's marriage to Edmée, establishes the long history between these women and Léa while at the same time introducing the latter to her newest foe. In the second episode, which features a menagerie of aging courtesans, Léa begins to see herself in the worn-out bodies of her old adversaries. Shot through with superficial compliments and catty commentary, both scenes reveal the vehement personal rivalries simmering just beneath the surface of these apparent friendships. Rather than portray the courtesan's world as an idyllic safe haven for feminine self-discovery, Colette exposes it as a fierce arena of feminine confinement and conflict.

The courtesan's world, as the first parlor scene so expertly divulges, was, above all, an incessantly rotating kaleidoscope of appearances. Beneath the artificial valance of camaraderie—the quaint domestic setting, the seemingly polite exchange of pleasantries, a meeting intended to affably unite two houses—Charlotte, Marie-Laure, and Léa ruthlessly evaluate one another. The façade of friendship enables them to settle the business of marriage, but it does not successfully mask their latent animosities. Introducing the hostess as a "dimpled nymph" with "implacable eyes, the delicate aggressive nose, and a still coquettish way of standing with her feet in fifth position" (18), the narrator sets the scene by demonstrating how even innocuous observations could be transformed into scathing insults. On the one hand, Charlotte resembles a delicately nosed, coquettish nymph still capable of attracting sexual attention despite her age. On the other, she appears "implacable," "aggressive" and ridiculous in her insistence on recalling her long bygone days as a dancer.

The duplicity of the courtesan's world is further echoed in descriptions of Marie-Laure, a lifelong rival to both Charlotte and Léa. As Marie-Laure enters the parlor with her adolescent daughter, Léa greets her insincerely as "perfection itself" (19). The narrator interjects, describing Marie-Laure as a "red-haired young woman with brown eyes, whose physical presence was enough to take your breath away." But even the narrator cannot resist adding that "she drew attention, almost coquettishly," an observation that renders double-edged Léa's remark that "Marie-Laure alters only to become always more disconcertingly lovely" (19). Chéri, too, cannot prevent himself from offering his own snide commentary. "That woman," he thinks to himself of his future mother-in-law, "must have a dozen corpses in her wake. Dolled up in jade green, red hair, painted to look eighteen, and the inevitable smile" (44). It is through her critique of Marie-Laure, moreover, that Léa's first impression of her daughter, Chéri's future wife, Edmée, materializes. "She's just the daughter for Marie-Laure," thought Léa, gazing at her more closely. "She has all her mother's dazzling qualities but in a quieter key: fluffy, ash-brown hair, that looks as if it were powdered, frightened, secretive eyes and a mouth she avoids opening even to speak or smile. . . . Exactly what Marie-Laure needs as a foil—but she must hate her!" (19). Assuming a rivalry between mother and daughter, Léa acknowledges beauty's centrality to the female self as well as its power to mercilessly position all women, despite their relation to one another, as enemies.

Depicting a casual afternoon of visiting and card playing, the second parlor scene illustrates how animosities persist among the courtesans even as they approach old age. Although once highly desirable, the minor characters introduced in this scene—the Baroness de la Berche, Madame Aldonza, and Lili—have not been nearly so well-preserved as Léa or Marie-Laure. "Madame Aldonza, an aged ballerina, with legs eternally swathed in bandages, was distorted with rheumatism," explains the narrator, "and wore her shiny black wig a little askew. Opposite her, a head or more taller, the Baroness squared her rigid shoulders like a country priest's. Her face was large and had grown alarmingly masculine with age. She was a bristling bush of hair—hair in her ears, tufts in her nostrils and on her lip, and rough hairs between her fingers." (48) Age has inflicted irreversible wounds upon Madame Aldonza, who, "distorted with rheumatism" and "swathed in bandages," suffers a permanently damaged, broken body. Though her body remains intact, covered with "bristling" hair and crowned by a large face that had grown "alarmingly masculine," the baroness has not fared much better. To make matters worse, Madame Aldonza and the Baroness de la Berche have not only lost their youth and beauty; they have also lost their femininity.[10]

Unlike Léa, for whom such loss posed a fate worse than death, Aldonza and Berche accept this new stage of life. As the scholar Martina Sternberger argues, these women undergo a "masculinizing metamorphosis" in which their "physical and phantasmatic 'virilization' . . . constitutes a zone of protection. . . . The capacity for dealing with historical and biological time is, in Colette's texts, an essentially 'female' aptitude—even if it paradoxically includes the capacity of 'de-femininizing' oneself in time."[11] For Sternberger, Colette's prostitutes extend the range of female possibilities and embody, in their ability to come to grips with their aging bodies, "a kind of avant-garde of female happiness"[12] Certainly, Sternberger's analysis helps explain how characters like Aldonza and Berche survive the advance of old age, but what about those characters who continued to resist the inevitability of aging?

Whereas Madame Aldonza and the Baroness de la Berche embrace retirement, the grotesque Lili insists on plying her trade despite her advanced age and expanding waistline. Loudly announcing her entry into Charlotte Peloux's parlor, the geriatric Lili eagerly shows off her latest adolescent lover. Léa carefully considers the spectacle:

> Perhaps seventy years of age, with the corpulence of a eunuch held in by stays, old Lili was usually referred to as "passing all bounds," without those "bounds" being defined. Her round pink painted face was enlivened by a ceaseless girlish gaiety, and her large eyes and small mouth, thin-lipped and shrunken, flirted shamelessly. Old Lili followed the fashion to an outrageous degree. A striking blue-and-white striped skirt held in the lower part of her body, and a little blue jersey gaped over her skinny bosom crinkled like the wattles of a turkey-cock; a silver fox failed to conceal the neck, which was the shape of a flower-pot and the size of a belly. (50)

Unable to tear her eyes away from Lili's body, Léa concludes that the older woman's appearance is "effroyable" (terrifying). Lili's body is frightening because she tries too hard to make it appear young and beautiful. Léa notes how absurd a "round pink painted face" animated by "ceaseless girlish gaiety" looks on a woman of seventy. Despite her most vigilant efforts, Lili could not escape her age; her "small mouth, thin-lipped and shrunken," could not be hidden even when it "flirted shamelessly," nor could her "skinny bosom crinkled like the wattles of a turkey-cock" be covered over by the latest fashions. For Léa, Lili's monstrous figure offers a scathing indictment of women who try too desperately to outlive and overuse their "well-made" bodies.

But must Lili's tragedy be the fate of all women who lived by their beauty? Lying in bed that evening, Léa considers the other women in the parlor. "Which of them am I going to look like in ten years' time?" she wonders (54). Rising in the middle of the night from a fitful sleep, she bathes her teary eyes, applies a coat of powder to her face, and then returns to bed. "She was on her guard, full of mistrust for an enemy she had never known: grief. She had just said goodbye to thirty years of easy living: years spent pleasantly, intent often on love, sometimes on money. This had left her, at almost fifty, still young and defenseless" (55). Léa realizes that losing her best physical assets would mean a marked decrease in her market value at the same time that it undermined her self-worth. For a woman whose identity had always resided in her beauty, the ravages of aging severely jeopardized how she valued herself as both a woman and an individual.

Ever resilient, Léa sets aside her fears of growing into an absurd, used-up old courtesan by turning to artifice to resurrect her youthful body. Léa has long congratulated herself for escaping the "elderly lechers" who so frequently find satisfaction in the courtesan's arms, and as she contemplates how to mask the signs of age appearing on her own body, she renews her resolve never to share her bed with "an old man of forty." Almost instinctively she "polishes her nails" before inspecting "the disastrous red of her hair with its graying roots" (95). In a moment of "moral indigestion" that oscillates between melancholy and panic, Léa attacks her roots, hoping to resurrect her youthful body. "She even thought of doing her hair differently; for twenty years she had worn it high, brushed straight off the neck. 'Rolled in curls low on the neck, like Lavalière? Then I should be able to cope with this year's loose-waisted dresses. With a strict diet, in fact, and my hair properly hennaed, I can hope for ten—no, let's say five years'" (95). Desperate to salvage her aging body and rejuvenated by fantasies of self-recovery, Léa works diligently to ensure that she will not become Lili.

Sporting newly dyed red hair, Léa attempts to rejoin the world that she knew before Chéri. Venturing out to the theater, where old male friends solicit her; to the boxing arena, where she endeavors unsuccessfully to reunite with former flames; to dinners, where young women greet her with deference, and traipsing across southern France trying out new lovers—Léa discovers that despite her efforts, Madame Peloux's parlor is where she most belongs. After a comfortable visit with her old friend, Léa "mused over her future, veering between alarm and resignation" (103). She contemplated her "fast approaching old age" and decided that maintaining her spirited rivalry with Charlotte Peloux, embracing the conflict of the woman's world, will spare her. She would become like the others, the "women past their prime, who abandon first their stays, then their hair dye, and who finally no longer bother about the quality of their underclothes" (103). Resigned to the life of the mature woman, Léa symbolically alternates her tea gowns with heavy boots and woolen jackets. Adorned in matronly attire, she escapes the notice of male passersby. Aligning herself with the Aldonzas and Berches rather than the Lilis of her set, Léa "faced this new life with the patience of an apprentice," determined to make peace with her aging body (104).

THE END OF BEAUTY?: LÉA AFTER CHÉRI

Léa's resolve is compromised, however, when late one night while lingering at her dressing table, combing and tugging at "hair stiffened by dye," she is startled by a noise outside her window (108). Before responding, "with an instinctive movement of self-preservation and modesty," Léa "ran to powder her face" (108). As she fortifies herself at her dressing table, Chéri barges into her bedroom. Upon seeing him after six months of separation, Léa so successfully steeled herself against his onslaught that she "felt at first only the resentment of a woman caught at her toilette." Anchored to her dressing table, Léa uses the toilette as a first line of defense against the intruder. Preparing herself for the impending conflict, Léa grabs for her powder in one "instinctive movement." Once she collects herself, she reprimands Chéri for his poor manners (108). Exasperated by Léa's cool response—she calmly buffs her nails while he fidgets in despair—Chéri begins overturning furniture and throwing off his clothes. Through the bedroom mirror Léa watches as he vents his frustration, accusing her of sharing herself with other men. Refusing to counter his accusations, Léa "returned to her dressing table, smoothed her hair, rearranged her comb, and, as if for want of something better to do, began unscrewing the top of a scent bottle" (111).

Momentarily protected, Léa turns to her cosmetics to conceal her nervousness—she feels vulnerable beneath Chéri's gaze and to maintain her indomitable façade, she masks her expression with powder and covers over her anxiety with nail polish. The ruse works, and Chéri, crushed by what he interprets as Léa's indifference, crumbles hysterically into her lap. At this, Léa can no longer restrain herself. She dislodges herself from her dressing table to comfort him. Eliciting from him an apology and a confession of love, Léa nestles Chéri in her arms like the "'naughty little boy' never born to her" (118). Confronted with the "presumptuous brutality of love," Léa abandons "the well-ordered prudence, the happy common sense that had been her guide through life, the humiliating vagaries of her riper years and the subsequent renunciations" (116).

Feigning sleep the next morning, Chéri gazes on his lover through slightly parted eyelashes. Breaking with her old routine, Léa headed first not for the looking glass but for the railway timetable. "Not yet powdered, a meager twist of hair at the back of her head, double chin, and raddled neck, she was exposing herself rashly to the unseen observer" (122). For the first time in their affair, Léa feels secure enough that she "forgets to perform, rashly exposing her aging body to his critical spectatorship."[13] Chéri watches as she happily moves about the boudoir and its adjoining rooms until, moderately disgusted and overcome with guilt for his spying, he finally pulls himself out of bed. When Léa returns to the bedroom, he is relieved to see her hair done and makeup on. Though Léa comfortably reveals her natural body to Chéri, it is not until after she has done her hair and touched up her face that he feels at ease with her. Ironically, it is at the very moment that Léa allows herself to become vulnerable that she loses her lover: for it is not Léa herself, but Léa the image that Chéri loves.

Initially oblivious to this loss, Léa enthusiastically explains how the couple will flee Paris. She reverts to old habits, plying Chéri with rhubarb tablets and hot chocolate. Chéri listens in silence, but unlike on previous occasions, he holds his tongue out of frustration rather than deference. Chéri reaches his boiling point, however, when Léa, noting his morose expression, condescendingly likens him to a prepubescent boy. He startles her by retorting, "Being with you Nounoune, is likely to keep me twelve for half a century" (127). As Léa exposed her aging, imperfect face to Chéri, he now shows his maturing self to her. Though Léa believed upon waking that Chéri was not a "passing fancy" but the great love of her life, when he asserts his independence, she realizes that she is not in love with Chéri himself but with her idea of Chéri.

"Love creates roles for Léa and Chéri," the critic Victoria Best points out, "at the same time as it destroys them, placing them in an identity relation of such mutual dependence that a change in their relationship results in a total collapse of their performances"[14] Léa has grown old, Chéri has started to grow up, and, in the process, both have tired of producing the ideal, the somebody else that the other so desired.

This role reversal proves Léa's undoing. "You came back," she whispers, "and find an old woman." Holding Chéri, Léa asks, "At the age when a woman's life is so often over, was I really the loveliest for you, the most kind, and were you really in love with me?" (127). As she utters this question she suddenly understands the ludicrousness of a future with her young lover. "Go back to your youth and to your life," she tells him; "go back to a woman who will tremble with passion and not from the perverted mother-love" (129). As Chéri's lover, Léa indulged in fantasies of eternal youth; by giving him up, Léa puts aside the frivolities of youth and chooses sagacity over ridiculousness.

Léa's struggle for self-definition begins and ends with mastering her "well-made" body. Beauty distinguishes her from other women, it binds her to her young lover, and it shapes, in every way, how she experiences life as both a woman and an individual. Despite its centrality to Léa's identity in the novel, however, beauty was not a pivotal component of the original story. Serialized under the title "Clouk" in *Le matin* between 1911 and 1912, the first version of the story portrayed Léa not as a breathtaking enchantress but a plump old woman with white hair and loose flesh. Chéri (named Clouk) is himself an unattractive teenager addicted to drugs and abusive mistresses.[15] As in the novel, each lover idolizes a particular image of the other—Léa is drawn to Clouk's recklessness, and he is enamored with her monstrous body. Clouk first encounters Léa sitting at "the table with old ladies," finding her "overripe, enormous, and magnificent as a heavy fruit fallen beneath a tree."[16] Clouk desires to "slip over to their table, all frail and small, squeeze between those fat gossips' arms, amid the rustling skirts and the doughy knees, and lean up against the ample shoulders, lost, drowned in that melting warmth of slightly senile nannies."[17] Thus, in the initial rendition of the story it is the beauty of the grotesque that attracts Clouk and Léa.

But why, when she revised these short stories into a novel some eight years after their periodical début, would Colette completely reimagine her primary characters? Why transform the obscene into the beautiful? Reflecting on this issue, Colette explained her decision to recast Chéri this way:

> When I gave birth to this beautiful young man—who would believe it?—he was ugly, something of a runt, and sickly, suffering from swollen adenoids. But I had a feeling, that I would not form any attachment to this quasi-scrofulous child. Spurned and thin-skinned, Clouk awoke from a few months' sleep, cast off his pale little slough like a molting snake, emerged gleaming, devilish, unrecognizable, and I wrote the first version of *Chéri* without knowing at the time that a few succinct, casual stories would ripen and grow into rather bitter novels.[18]

Perhaps it was Colette's inability to "form any attachment to this quasi-scrofulous child" that made Chéri's beauty necessary. But what was the rationale behind re-creating Léa as well? Why not permit her to remain "overripe, enormous, and magnificent"? By making Léa beautiful, Colette not only made her Chéri's physical equal; she also created a narrative space for analyzing how woman's aging body tipped the scales balancing beauty and power.

For Léa, beauty and power are intimately intertwined. The courtesan's beautiful body enables her to dominate the opposite sex, to earn a comfortable income, and to live autonomously, free to pursue her own pleasures. As she ages, however, Léa confronts the reality that as her body declines so does her influence. Desperate to prolong the inevitable, Léa attempts to resurrect her fading beauty through Chéri's attractive body. As his mistress, she molds his body into an ideal physical specimen. Projecting her desire for eternal corporeal perfection onto Chéri's form, moreover, Léa uses his body as a distorted mirror—seeing reflected in it her own youth and beauty. Through his image and through his image of her, Chéri keeps Léa forever ageless and attractive. For Léa, then, ending the affair involved not only unraveling a romantic attachment but also coming face to face once and for all with the fragile woman hidden behind the "high-slung breasts," the "long legs and straight back," and the "well-made body" that had for so long enabled her to survive.

For the entirety of her adult life, beauty was Léa's only ambition. Léa used her "well-made" body to defy social norms, to attain financial independence, and ultimately to conquer the desirable Chéri. As Léa's aging body betrays her, however, she learns two difficult lessons simultaneously: first, that beauty is ephemeral and that its promises, like its powers, are fleeting; and second, that for the courtesan, who earns her living pleasing the opposite sex, a loss of beauty necessarily engenders a loss of power. Because Léa's body has power only as long as men continue to value it, losing her beauty means also acknowledging the degree to which she has allowed herself to be defined by and in relation to men. Colette herself cleverly foreshadowed this epiphany by entitling the novel not "Léa" or "The Courtesan," but *Chéri;* for Léa exists only as Chéri's lover, his surrogate mother, his ideal. Attached to Chéri in this way, Léa is incapable of imagining an identity beyond her "well-made" body, and she never fully achieves meaningful self-awareness. Chéri may have grown up in a woman's world, but Léa, like so many of the women who came of age in the 1890s, lives her entire life in the shadow of men.

ARTIFICIAL BEAUTY: RENÉE BEHIND THE MASK

Although confronted with many of the same challenges as Léa, the heroine of *La vagabonde,* Renée Néré, uses work to surmount the obstacle of the aging body. Like Léa, Renée is forced, at the end of a love affair, to assess her body, her beauty, and her place in the world. Renée's struggle is different from Léa's, however, because, unlike Léa, she eventually envisions an identity that is not confined to her beautiful body. Onstage, she produces an anonymous somebody else, performing an infinite range of fictions, all of which veil the "me" behind the mask.[19] In the mirror, she attempts to resolve the contradictions of her split personality through a series of repetitious acts, primarily applying and removing makeup. And in her letters she employs language to literally author a transcendent self. Although vastly different in form, each of these sites of self-production exposes the centrality of corporeal beauty to Renée's valuation of herself as both a woman and an individual.

A thirty-something music-hall performer struggling to reclaim her identity after a painful divorce while at the same time coming to terms with her aging body, Renée obsesses over her appearance. For Renée, the cosmetically enhanced body acts as a protective shell for her vulnerable, broken self. Applying makeup to transform her appearance for a role is crucial to Renée's self-recovery because it enables her to command not only the physical template of her body—through a disciplined beautification routine—but also to produce a intact, public self. By acting out a different fictive self each night, Renée uses her female body as "a canvas upon which identity displays are carefully created, by an act of self-conscious will."[20] Cosmetics, an integral part of Renée's performance, thus permit the actress to become somebody by temporarily playing at being somebody else.

Cosmetics facilitate Renée's appropriation of new stage identities at the same time that they safeguard her fragile ego. After a performance she glimpses herself in a backstage mirror and confesses how completely vulnerable she feels when out of character. Removing her grease paints, she extols: "There's no getting away from it, it really is me there behind that mask of purplish rouge, my eyes ringed with a halo of blue grease-paint beginning to melt. Can the rest of my face be going to melt also? What if nothing were to remain from my whole reflection but a streak of dyed color stuck to the glass like a long, muddy tear?"[21] Afraid that what was once beautiful about her face might melt away and petrified that "it really is me there behind that mask," Renée acknowledges the intimate link between her physical appearance and her psychological well-being.

Almost sadistic in her attraction to her mirror, Renée searches it desperately for hidden truths. She is simultaneously relieved and unsatisfied to find that "what I see in the big looking-glass in my bedroom is no longer the painted image of an itinerant music-hall artiste. It reflects only—myself" (11). Under intense scrutiny, Renée's face reveals all that is inadequate in her life: "Alone, alone, and for the rest of my life, no doubt. Already alone; it's early for that. When I turned thirty I did not feel cast down because mine is a face that depends on the expression which animates it, the color of my eyes, and the defiant smile that plays over it" (11). Mourning the loss of the "color" of her eyes, longing to reclaim that "defiant smile" of her youth, Renée barely recognizes the face of the woman peering back at her.

Unable to fully comprehend this revelation, Renée attempts to see herself through the eyes of others, particularly the objectifying gaze of her male colleagues. Focusing on the smile that Marinetti called her *gaiezza volpina* and on her lips that, according to her theater partner Brague, make her face look pinched like a rat's, she finds familiarity as well as disappointment in this experiment. From their criticisms, which she has memorized and internalized, she levels her own:

> But how I dislike seeing myself with that drooping mouth and those slack shoulders, the weight of my whole sad body slumped on one leg! My hair hangs dank and lank and in a little while I shall have to brush its shining beaver brown. My eyes are still faintly ringed with blue eye-shadow and there's a wavering trace of red on my nails. It will take me at least fifty good minutes of bathing and grooming to get rid of all that. (12)

The "drooping mouth," "slack shoulders," and hair "dank and lank" signify Renée's aging body as well as her forlorn psychological state. That there is nothing firm, certain, or positive in Renée's body language reflects her lack of self-confidence, while the remnants of faint "blue eye-shadow" and the "trace of red" on her nails signify her marginal profession and echo the precariousness of her place in the world. Caught in a transitional moment between stage performance and self performance, moreover, Renée confronts her loneliness, understanding well that it will take much more than "fifty good minutes of bathing and grooming to get rid of all that."

Colette lucidly articulates Renée's discomfort with her social alienation by explaining the actress's anxiety before performing in the home of a bourgeois society woman. Fifteen minutes prior to taking center stage in the parlor, Renée confides: "I look at myself in the mirror and find myself ugly, deprived of the harsh electric-light which, in my dressing-room, floods the white walls, bathes the mirrors, penetrates one's make-up and gives it a velvety look" (57). In the music hall, a contrived public space, Renée performs at a safe distance from the audience, and she is protected behind the theater's atmosphere of masquerade. In this realm, she derives identity from that which is external—she is an image caught in the crowd's singular, undifferentiated gaze. Onstage, completely divorced from her personal identity, Renée is an anonymous spectacle, a figment, a character who exists entirely independently of the woman who embodies her. However, in a private home, the bastion of domesticity no less, without the lighting, the stage, and the magic of the theater, Renée becomes visible and knowable to her audience. In this scenario, makeup merely provides a mask that inadequately disguises the woman whom everybody already knows. In this mirror, then, Renée sees herself not as an illusory artiste but as a gross caricature of the women she once was.

Renée's fascination with her own reflection, especially at moments when she is quite literally between selves, is indicative of her vagabondage. Her wondering mind signifies her wandering self and becomes an almost narcissistic fixation. Moreover, her scopophilic preoccupation with her body,[22] the sexual response she elicits from looking at her physical form, does not incite pleasure in the self but functions to resurrect her lost subjectivity.[23] Renée's narcissism, her fixation on loving the self as an image (the ego ideal), provides the foundation for her subjectivity at the same time that it ensures that she remain alienated from her genuine self. In the above scenes, Colette shows how Renée uses cosmetics to cover over her damaged self while at the same time attempting to reproduce a new one.[24] The ritual of putting on and removing her makeup, in this context, symbolizes the constant tug-of-war within her. Involving strict bodily discipline, for Renée the contest for self-definition plays out in a deeply corporeal way.

Throughout these scenes, Renée maneuvers delicate imbrications of power and beauty. Initially Renée's power resides explicitly in her ability to master her body. By creating her physical body as an alluring spectacle, Renée succeeds as a stage performer at the same time that she constructs barriers that protect her from sincere human engagement. In the music hall, Renée gains financial independence at the expense of social intimacy. The hardworking colleagues with whom she shares the stage, while industrious and even enjoyable, prove no substitute for genuine attachments and meaningful affective bonds. As a stage performer, Renée precariously straddles two worlds and must constantly negotiate competing notions of who really is "there behind that mask."

CONTESTED BEAUTY: RENÉE AND MAX

Similar dislocations of self frame the novel's romance plot, which unfolds through a series of power plays between the protagonist and her persistent suitor—Maxime Dufferin-Chautel. Resigned to a life of solitude after ex-husband Taillandy's deceptions, Renée actively retreats from love, hiding behind her cosmetics and her stage personas, desperate to protect herself from future heartache. Despite taking extreme precautions, however, Renée finds herself pursued relentlessly. On their first meeting, Max invades her dressing room, awkwardly declaring his affections, sending her flowers, and obviously regarding her as little more than an object of desire. Annoyed by his clumsy overtures, Renée playfully designates him the "Le Grand Serin" (a derogatory nickname that translates imperfectly as the "big dope"), and, satisfied that he will soon relent, she aggressively defends herself against his advances.

Undeterred by Renée's lack of interest, Max persists in his campaign, orchestrating meetings and attempting to woo her with trinkets until she reluctantly warms to him: "His belief in me, the innocent belief of a man very much in love, enlightened me about myself that evening just as an unexpected mirror, at a street corner or on a staircase, suddenly reveals blemishes and sagging in one's face and figure" (106). Comparing Max to a mirror, Renée enters dangerous territory, for now she sees her reflection not in a piece of glass but through the eyes of a lover. Although Max incessantly praises her appearance, Renée nevertheless compares his gaze to a cruel mirror that "reveals blemishes and sagging in one's face and figure." Under Max's gaze, Renée surrenders herself, admitting, "I 'let myself go' . . . mouth tired and shut and eyes deliberately dull, and to my admirer's persistence I oppose the passive bearing of a girl whom her parents want to marry against her will" (107). Renée's physical body, her "mouth tired and shut" and her "eyes deliberately dull," signifies her complete submission to Max—an especially perilous move for a woman whose personhood is so intimately tied to the visual illusion she hides behind.

Although Renée capitulates to Max's attentions, she continues to cling to her makeup as a tool of self-preservation. Renée's preoccupation with her appearance protects her precisely because it confounds Max: "Whoever d'you want to put powder on for, at this hour?" he asks as the two share an evening alone. To which she replies, "For myself, in the first place. And then for you." (150). At the same time that Renée instinctively relies on her makeup for protection, she admits that her cosmetically enhanced face might prove more pleasing to her lover than her bare, natural one. Here cosmetics perform double duty by enabling Renée to conserve the fragile somebody so deliberately obscured behind the façade of the somebody else on the one hand, while making visible her desperate desire to please another on the other.

As the bond between the lovers grows, Renée increasingly finds herself uncomfortably caught between two competing identities. Desirous to see herself with her own eyes, on an outing with Max, she begins groping, with an anxious hand, for the looking glass in her little bag. When Max asks if she has lost something, she replies negatively and focuses attention away from herself. Despite her denial, in this moment, Renée begins to realize that she has indeed lost something—she has literally and figuratively lost sight of herself. This sense of loss is reiterated in a later episode, when Blandine, her charwoman, announces Max's arrival, and Renée frantically shuts herself into her room: "He musn't see my face! Quick! The rice powder, the kohl, the mascara . . . oh! You have aged!" (200). Desperate to conceal her imperfections from her suitor, she finally descends and is met with Max's exclamation, "'There you are at last, my darling, my scented one, my appetizing one, my . . ." (200). Tellingly, it is what is most artificial about Renée, her scent in this instance, that Max finds most "appetizing." Ironically, the same weapons that Renée relies upon for protection, grease paints on her face and scented lotions permeating her skin, also map Max's colonization of her body.

Renée's preoccupation with her aging body and her recognition that Max has eroded her defenses leaves her profoundly unsettled. She writes to him in a letter:

> Are not the things you love in me the things which change me and deceive you, my curls clustering thick as leaves, my eyes which the blue kohl lengthens and suffuses, the artificial smoothness of my powdered skin? What would you say if I were to reappear before you with my heavy, straight hair, with my fair lashes cleansed of their mascara, in short with the eyes which my mother gave me, crowned with brief eyebrows quick to frown, grey, narrow, level eyes in the depths of which there shines a stern, swift glance which I recognize as that of my father? (258)

Convinced that Max's love for her is based entirely on her appearance, Renée challenges his admiration for her "clustering thick" curls, her eyes lengthened with blue kohl, and the "artificial smoothness" of her powdered skin. Renée gave her youth to the treacherous Taillandy, and she believes that her fading beauty will not be enough to keep Max, who will love neither her "heavy, straight hair" nor her "fair lashes cleansed of their mascara." It was, after all, Taillandy's inability to appreciate the real Renée that led to his infidelities and to her vagabondage. And, as Renée knows well, in a culture that values youth, an attractive aging body is even more flawed than an imperfect, young one. Thus the contest between Max and Renée is not only over possession of her beautiful body but also for power over her identity as a woman.

When Renée enters into the relationship with Max, her power emanates primarily from his appraisal of her body. Seduced by her corporeal beauty, in love with both her appearance and the idea of her, Max initially submits to playing by Renée's rules. Although she learns quickly that she can use her body to extract material objects from him, by making Max her lover, Renée risks her heart. If she gives herself to him, as she had given herself to Taillandy, she understands that she will necessarily cede power. She attempts to prevent this loss by continuing to control her appearance—groping for her looking glass, powdering her face—but she is unable to fully accomplish this task because Max constantly interrupts her efforts with his "Whoever d'you want to put powder on for, at this hour?" Through his unintentionally disruptive acts, Max, the big dope, skillfully disarms Renée, offering her stability, social acceptance, and comfort all at the cost of her personal liberation.

TRANSIENT BEAUTY: VICTORIES AND VAGABONDS

In a series of letters to Max, Renée confesses her unvoiced insecurities and uses the act of writing as a cathartic release for coming to terms with her fading beauty. In print, these anxieties become yet another mirror through which Renée contemplates her identity as an aging woman. Significantly, it is through this process of critical self-appraisal that Renée finds the courage to disengage from Max. "It is not suspicion, not your future betrayal, my love, which is devastating me, it is my own inadequacy." Renée is inadequate because she cannot stop the passage of time. She explains, "We are the same age; I am no longer a young woman. Oh my love, imagine yourself in a few years' time, as a handsome man in the fullness of your age, beside me in mine! Imagine me, still beautiful but desperate, frantic in my armor of corset and frock, under my make-up and powder, in my young, tender colors" (296–97). Because her body has deceived her, made her older and thus unable to compete with youthful beauties, Renée retreats from Max, afraid that his repulsion of her naturally aging body will inexorably lead to betrayal and suffering (301).

Confiding her anxieties in these letters permits Renée to finally confront her aging body: "Everything is against me. The first obstacle I run into is the female body lying there, which bats my way, a voluptuous body with closed eyes, deliberately blind, stretched out and ready to perish rather than leave the place where its joy lies. That woman there, that brute bent on pleasure, is I myself" (301–2). No longer "deliberately blind," Renée acknowledges that, as a "brute bent on pleasure," she has relinquished her personal autonomy to men. As Renée learns to accept her natural body, she also begins to reconcile the many selves warring beneath its surface. Still fearful of solitude, she nevertheless chooses to go it alone: "Max, my well-beloved adversary, how will lacerating myself help me to get the better of you? You would only have to appear and . . . But I am not calling to you to come! . . . No, I am not calling to you to come. It is my first victory" (302). Renée's victory lies not only in refusing to submit to Max, but also in the recovery of her self—in rescuing the somebody rather than merely accommodating the somebody else.

In the final part of the novel, Renée endeavors to reclaim that part of herself which Max has taken away. She knows that to enjoy full sovereignty she must sever ties with her lover and extricate herself from the bourgeois world he inhabits. Once again, her beauty acts as friend and foe. Still attractive and able to portray countless characters on stage, Renée continues to pursue a career based on appearances and performance—a career that releases her from Max and enables her to rebuild the protective wall around her fragile ego that he has started to dismantle. Yet for Renée, self-preservation comes at the ultimate price: embracing the solitary adventure of the vagabond, she could very easily find herself "alone! alone and for the rest of [her] life, no doubt" (10).

Married to Taillandy, Renée embodied the domestic ideal—she served as her husband's decorative foible, and, as a good bourgeois, she kept up appearances, never transgressing social norms or revealing the indiscretions of her husband. In this capacity, Renée embraced a self that was safely conventional, vacuously respectable, and painfully incomplete. In his desire to have Renée as his own kept woman, Max offers her a similarly stable and limited life. As a vagabond, in search of the "real me" behind the mask, Renée chooses self-love over love for others. Renée's conversion is tentative, even agonizing as she schizophrenically oscillates between one self and another. Divorcing romantic love from love of self, desiring to matter not to others but to oneself, and choosing the somebody over the somebody else, Renée emerges in Colette's novel as a liberated, if lonely, New Woman. Through Renée's vagabondage, then, Colette opens a space for imagining a multiplicity of female experiences. In so doing, she suggests that there is more than one way to become somebody, more than one route to becoming a woman.

Although Colette ended *La vagabonde* with Renée's ambivalent departure into eternal vagabondage, that is not how she finished Renée's story. In her sequel to the novel entitled *L'entrave* (*The Shackle*), Colette picks up Renée's story three years later. During the time that has passed, the protagonist has lost Hammond, Margot, and her dear animal avatar, Fosette, and she has retired from the music hall to live comfortably on a private income Margot bequeathed her. The novel opens with Renée's chance sighting of Max at the seaside. He is married and doting on his young child. After witnessing the scene, Renée retreats to her mirror demanding, "Have I aged? Yes, no, yes and no."[25] Moreover, it is as part of an ill-matched quartet—a twenty-five-year-old free spirit named May, her abusive, playboy boyfriend Jean, and the opium-addicted eccentric Masseau—that Renée has aged while managing to hold on to the vestiges of youth.

The peculiar dynamic of this group, interestingly, enables Renée to enjoy society while retaining her solitude. Indeed, the group dines together and goes on outings but shares little in the way of the confidences that mark the bonds of real friendship. The only intimacies May and Renée share, for example, involve discussions of the former's romantic skirmishes with Jean. The emotional distance between these women is made clear when May discloses one particularly charged argument as she performs her daily toilette. Rather than focus on what May is saying, Renée becomes absorbed in what she is doing. "By now her face was powdered mauve," Renée notices, "and touched with bright pink under the eyes that she had accentuated with grey eye shadow to make them look voluptuously heavy. Eyelashes . . . mouth . . . big velvet beauty spot at the corner of her mouth. It was finished." As Renée watches, May confides that Jean always criticized her regime, exclaiming, "What an ugly sight a pretty woman's toilette is!" Then why continue to carry it out in front of him? Renée inquires. "My dear!" May flippantly replies, "I don't say that when I'm thirty-five or forty, I won't hide when I do my face, but now! I haven't got pimples, have I? Or wrinkles, or red-rimmed eyes? Nothing to hide, anyone can have a good look at it! Either one's natural or one isn't" (46). May's comment coupled with Renée's role reversal (in *La vagabonde,* it was always Renée's toilette that was scrutinized) demonstrate that the great gulf separating these women is age. Although one of only three toilettes detailed in *L'entrave,* this scene, like those in *La vagabonde,* also positions characters within the narrative. Renée's voyeuristic attention to May's toilette signals her power over her younger companion. Like Max and the others who intruded into her actor's loge, Renée now makes woman the object of her gaze.

Renée's power position is short-lived, however, as she finds herself once more ensnared in the predatory gaze of man. This time it is Jean who catches her off-guard as she prepares herself for lunch. Renée narrates this second toilette scene: "I powdered my face and reddened my lips with the inefficient aid of a pocket mirror, too small to be of much use." As she reaches this conclusion, Jean interrupts her: "'The left cheek,' advised Jean, 'It has as much right to it as the other. Wipe your eyebrows. There!'" Renée, "secretly humiliated" by this encounter, assumes that "this morning he did not find me pretty, that he was comparing me with the Renée of Nice and I nervously responded by 'pulling together' my tired features." Her reaction, she assures herself, has nothing to do with Jean. "Any woman instinctively performs this defiant feat of facial gymnastics—which consists in faintly smiling to refine the shape of the lips, raising eyebrows, expanding the nostrils and tightening the muscles under the slightly slackening chin—even for the uninterested eye of a passing stranger" (92–93). Renée's humiliation signifies an acquiescence of power, the feminine surrender to the masculine that occurs under the spotlight of man's gaze.

Colette flips the script once more in the third and final toilette scene, which belongs to Jean. Renée and Jean abandon May to embark on their own affair. Once the two have consummated their union, Renée supervises her lover's toilette. "For the pleasure of following Jean and assisting at his toilette, I had stopped attending to my own," she confides. "And now I saw myself in a loose dressing gown, with my hair in becoming disorder. But my figure, beside the streamlined tails, the starched shirt front, the pale, clean-shaven face, looked sluttish and untidy; there was a heaviness about it, an indefinable air of voluptuous maturity" (160). Renée has relinquished to Jean that which she could not give Max—as indicated in the heaviness of her body, the disheveled clothing and mussed hair, Renée has fully let herself go. As the older woman, Renée ministers to Jean in the same ways that Léa tends to Chéri, and in both cases it is age that establishes power within the relationship and that creates roles for the lovers.

Driven by an all-consuming need, Renée commits herself fully to her young lover. She agonizes over his feelings for her: "If he does not need me enough, what have I been doing all of this time and what future have I with him?" She admits, moreover, that "he is more necessary to me than air and water, I prefer him to the brittle possessions a woman calls her dignity or her self-esteem" (190–91). Renée's anxieties prove well-founded as, inevitably, Jean tires of his mature mistress and proposes that she go back to the stage, that she, in essence, return to her vagabondage. She tells him that she no longer has a profession, that she has given it up. Then, in a heartfelt aside, she explains to the reader how Jean has replaced her cherished *métier.* She confides: "There no longer exists any profession for me. There is only one aim in my life and it is there in front of me—this man who does not desire me and whom I love. To capture him . . . and recapture him . . . henceforth that is my only profession" (220). When Jean threatens to leave, Renée refuses to let *him* go. Through verbal and sexual manipulation, she manages to keep him shackled to her. In the last line of the novel, Renée's journey has come full circle: "It seems to me, as I watch him launch out enthusiastically into life, that he has changed places with me; that he is the eager vagabond and that I am the one who gazes after him, anchored forever" (224).

It is tempting to read this final admission as Renée's total and complete surrender. On the surface, she has renounced her independence to live as a man's mistress—the very fate that she resisted when she left Max at the end of the first book. Yet, closer examination suggests that although Renée relinquishes her vagabondage, she does not become merely a kept woman. Renée refused Max because of the life he offered; it is not domesticity that she wants so much as love. Certainly, with Jean she accepts the shackle of a monogamous, heterosexual union, but with him she also gets passion. As Melanie Collado argues, she finds "an actor and spectator to rival herself."[26] In this unconventional relationship she gets to play a role that is always changing, unstable, and never clearly scripted. In short, she gets to play a role worthy of an actress. Thus it is through struggle rather than through resolution that Renée comes to understand herself as a woman.

On New Year's Day 1909, Colette gazed into her hand mirror and discovered the first "claw marks" of age. Three weeks shy of her thirty-sixth birthday and still regarded as a charismatic Parisian treasure, she told herself, "You have to get old. . . . Repeat the words to yourself, not as a howl of despair but as the boarding call to a necessary departure"[27] As Colette contemplated her reflection, her life was at a crossroads. Her divorce from first husband, Willy, was imminent after three years of separation, her love affair with her mistress, Missy (Mathilde de Morney), was beginning to come undone, and, though she busied herself touring the country as a stage performer and by contributing articles to several newspapers and magazines, she felt utterly isolated and terribly alone. In 1910, Colette toured the provinces with the play *La chair*, and, away from Willy and Missy, she converted her makeup case into a makeshift writing table and began crafting the stories that would eventually become *Chéri* and *La vagabonde*.

Through Léa and Renée, Colette explored the murky politics of feminine self-production. Pursuing professions that valued superficiality over substance, the courtesan and the music-hall performer too easily conflated appearance with identity. Equating womanhood exclusively with the beautiful body, moreover, these characters focused for so long on preserving the artificial somebody else that they almost completely lost sight of the authentic somebody restlessly hovering in its shadow. For Léa and Renée, beauty poses the ultimate contradiction: on the one hand, because it is admired, it is a ticket to independence and pleasure; on the other, because it is fleeting, it is a passport to solitude and sadness. It is not until Léa and Renée wipe away the kohl, wash the dye out of their overdone hair—when they relinquish the performance of the beautiful woman—that they reassess how they viewed themselves *as* women. In the face of beauty, Léa and Renée could only play at being somebody else. In its absence, they learn that who they are as women emanates only in part from their "well-made" bodies.

Given their philosophical engagement with woman's struggle to create herself as an individual, reading *La vagabonde* and *Chéri* narrowly as melodramatic love stories or as imperfect facsimiles of Colette's real life overlooks their broader cultural relevance. Certainly, inasmuch as these novels problematize romantic love, they are romantic; and, inasmuch as Colette projected her own anxieties about woman's aging body onto her heroines, they might be considered autobiographical. The more enduring impact of these novels, however, resides in their portrayal of woman's struggle to reconcile beauty's promises and perils. The French New Woman, as she emerged in Colette's texts, cultivated a particular relationship to beauty. The stereotypical Anglo-Scandinavian New Woman was notable for her austerity as well as her audacity. Colette's New Woman, by contrast, preferred ostentation over modesty. The consummate performer, Renée could not give up the stage; while Léa, unable to cope with the matron's heavy boots and colorless tea gowns, continued to adorn her "well-made" body. Passionate, pleasure-seeking, and unapologetically preoccupied with appearances, Colette's protagonists, though exceptional, nevertheless resonated with audiences. *La vagabonde* was quickly turned into a play and then made into a film in 1916, and *Chéri,* which sold thirty thousand copies in the first six months after its debut in 1920, was made into a Hollywood feature film in 1950 and then again in 2009.

In her novels, Colette depicted beauty as a complex tour de force, a fluid category constantly under revision. For Colette, beauty was artificial, contested, transient, subversive, competitive, infinite and finite simultaneously. It posed more questions for women than it answered, and it rested at the center of how her characters understood themselves as both women and individuals. In light of her narrative obsession with the body beautiful, it should come as no surprise that Colette grappled with beauty's conundrums in her own life. How Colette struggled to resist the claw marks of age, to discipline her own well-made body, and to leave her mark on the beauty industry will be the focus of the next chapter.

4

Beauty and the Business of Becoming a Woman

To become nothing but a woman! It's not much, and yet
I threw myself toward this ordinary end.
—Colette, "Le Passé"

A publicity photograph from 1932 features a fully made-up, fashionably coiffed Colette adorned in a stylish, if conservative, black-and-white skirted business suit. Arms outstretched, gaze intense, focused, defiant, Colette exudes authority. Behind her, four white, wall-mounted shelves exhibit meticulously arranged black jars and clear glass bottles; below her, a glass-topped chrome table displays thirteen round white disks; above her, in the author's own scribbled script, looms the provocative question, "Are you for or against the writer's second career?" Filled with creams, lotions, and pomades, the containers in the photo were beauty products that Colette herself fabricated, packaged, and placed for sale inside her very own *institute de beauté*. In her fiction, Colette had long appreciated beauty's role in the process of feminine self-production; by launching a "second career" as the *directrice* of her own cosmetics company, she demonstrated that beauty work was more than a personal investment; it was a necessary labor, a partner indispensible to the work of becoming a woman.

By no means inevitable, Colette's foray into the beauty industry was not altogether unexpected. Industrious, unpredictable, appreciative of the merits of hard work, Colette shrewdly took advantage of the opportunities afforded her.[1] By the time that she opened her institute, Colette had not only established herself as one of France's most celebrated authors, but she had also conquered two of the most dynamic culture industries of the early twentieth century—the stage and the press. Offering paid work, a forum for self-expression, and public visibility, theater and journalism, as Mary Louise Roberts has shown, proved "empowering worlds for women."[2] Colette used these worlds not only to secure her own financial independence, but also to advance a model of womanhood that championed self-development and self-fulfillment.[3] Moreover, by capitalizing on all that the city of Paris offered—a vibrant print culture that routinely served up fantasies of the self, a theatrical urban landscape that blurred fiction and reality, and a flourishing consumer market[4]—Colette used creative work to expand the repertoire of acceptable social and professional roles for women. In light of Colette's activities, her entrée into the beauty industry should not be read, as it was by many of her contemporaries and has been by several scholars since, as a peculiar diversion or an ill-conceived feminine whim; rather, it should be understood as a logical progression, a culmination of her lifelong efforts to reconcile work, beauty, and womanhood.

This chapter shifts focus onto some of Colette's less-studied works, exploring her essays devoted to the behind-the-scenes experiences of music-hall performers, her journalistic writings about quotidian engagements with beauty and fashion, and the interviews and publicity materials that accompanied the launch of her cosmetics firm, to show how Colette attempted to square beauty and work with womanhood. In each of these writings, makeup reveals the intimate, casting light on the private relationships and experiences that govern daily life. It signals as well the transitory and the transformative, illuminating the myriad ways that femininity is performed in rhythm with the fast pace of modern life. Finally, it illustrates the hard work, the constant effort required to succeed in the ordinary business of becoming a woman.

BEAUTY IN THE MUSIC HALL: PERFORMING THE "USUALLY SCATTERED SELF"

In a letter to her close friend, the actress and poet Hélène Picard, Colette confessed her too frequent inability to harness her "usually scattered self."[5] It is not altogether surprising that Colette, a woman who so convincingly embodied countless personas on the music-hall stage, should struggle to keep track of her self in her real life. Through her skillful role playing, both onstage and off—appearing publicly in drag, personifying characters from her own stories, posing as a devoted wife or mistress, acting the part of the intellectual one moment, the ingénue the next—Colette intentionally invited misidentifications that made it difficult for even the performer herself to always recognize the woman hidden "there behind that mask."

Embodying an infinite array of (primarily female) characters onstage, Colette came to appreciate the many ways that femininity was constructed through appearance via cosmetics and fashion and through comportment via language and gesture. She explored the fluidity of identity not only through stage performance but also in a series of short stories that she authored during her career. Semiautobiographical, these stories meticulously revealed the mundane details of music-hall life and labor. Colette vividly recounted the daily trials of her colleagues, both real and imagined, privileging, at every turn, the underbelly of show-business glamour. In the music hall and in her writings about it, Colette explored the central paradox of stage performance, the tension between hard work (the hidden, grueling labor required to execute the spectacle) and effortless beauty (the public, artistic expression that unfolds to audiences during the performance itself).

In all of her writings devoted to the music hall, Colette drew heavily on her own experiences as an actress. She entered the profession as her marriage to first husband, Willy, unraveled, and she took her job seriously from the outset, regarding it as a skill to be learned and a craft to be mastered.[6] In 1905, she began taking lessons from the esteemed Georges Wague, a talented mime with whom she would perform throughout her tenure. Alongside Wague, Colette made her professional début at the Théâtre des Mathurins on February 6, 1906, playing the lead in *L'amour, le desir, la chimère,* a pantomime by Francis de Croisset and Jean Nougués. Between 1906 and 1913, the pair headlined hundreds of productions across France, Belgium, and Switzerland.[7] Colette proved herself a talented performer and a shrewd businesswoman, explaining to Wague as early as 1909 that her name had already "proved its box office value." Like Sarah Bernhardt before her, Colette negotiated the terms of her theater contracts, but she also went further, managing her own publicity by sending photos of herself to magazine editors with precise instructions for captions and placement.[8]

In addition to performing with Wague, Colette appeared in stage versions of her own works. In 1909, she starred in Willy's adaptation of *Claudine à Paris* and then in her own play, *En comrades.* She left the tour in 1911 to return to Paris not to embody Judith or Venus, but to star as Renée Néré. Even after unofficially retiring from the stage, Colette was often drawn back to the theater to portray her most celebrated heroines. In February 1922, Colette played Léa in the one-hundredth stage performance of *Chéri*—a role she would reprise numerous times over the next four years—and in 1927, she headlined once more as France's most recognizable, most exquisitely tortured vagabond.[9] At the height of her celebrity, Colette's image became so imbricated with her characters that when Pierre Drieu La Rochelle spotted the kohl-rimmed eyes of a woman walking her little dog in Paris's seventh arrondissement, he immediately exclaimed, "It's the Vagabond!"[10]

Colette chronicled her impressions of music-hall life, most notably, of course, in *La vagabonde,* but also in a series of short stories, published originally in *Le matin* and then collected in 1913 under the title *Music Hall Sidelights* (*L'envers du music hall*). In these stories, Colette offered readers a backstage pass, a behind-the-scenes glimpse into the real-life experiences of stage performers that audiences rarely had the privilege of witnessing firsthand. Focusing on the quotidian and the banal, Colette humanized performers and portrayed music-hall life as economically precarious, physically strenuous, mentally arduous, and emotionally exhausting. She sensitively articulated the performer's daily struggles by highlighting his/her engagement with ordinary stage props: cosmetics, costumes, and undergarments. Four of the twenty-three stories in *L'envers,* in fact, recounted backstage experiences explicitly through the lens of stage makeup. In "The Halt," "The Workroom," "Matinee," and "Love," makeup acts as an equal player in the narrative: it sets the scene; it defines characters; it even expresses emotion. More than any other tool of the trade, makeup, for Colette, reveals the hidden world of the music-hall artiste, casting light on her talents and shortcomings, her pragmatism and vanity, her mask and the scattered selves warring just beneath its surface.

In "The Halt," makeup, or rather its remnants, communicates the hardships of life on the road. Exhausted and disheveled, the touring actors arrive at a small-town train station, "an ugly lot, graceless, and lacking humility: pale from too-hard work, or flushed after a hastily snatched lunch. . . . Trailing over the length and breadth of France, we have slept in our crumpled bonnets."[11] The one exception in this motley crew appears to be the "*grande coquette,* above whose head wave pompously—stuck on the top of a dusty black velvet tray—three funeral ostrich plumes" (106). Upon closer inspection, however, not even the coquette escapes the uncomfortable voyage unscathed. Despite her efforts to appear composed, sporting "carefully waved tresses of . . . peroxide hair," she has neglected to fully eliminate the evidence of her previous engagement. As the wind blows back her hat, the narrator notices that "across her forehead—between eyebrows and hair—a carelessly removed red line, the trace of last night's makeup" (106). Thus even the audacious ostrich feathers fail to mask what the carelessly expunged makeup exposes: the coquette is every bit as weary and overworked as the other members of her troupe.

After critiquing her colleague, the narrator turns a critical eye to her own tousled appearance. Inspecting her reflection in a watchmaker's storefront window, she laments her own "shimmerless hair" and criticizes "the sad twin shadows under my eyes, lips parched with thirst," before denouncing her "flabby figure" (106). Suffering from the same fatigue as her compatriots, the narrator acknowledges the toll that unremitting physical exertion and too many late nights has exacted. Comparing herself disparagingly to a "discouraged beetle," a "molting bird," and a "governess in distress," she concludes matter-of-factly, "Good Lord, I look like an actress on tour and that speaks for itself" (106). Through the narrator's ridicule of both herself and her colleagues, Colette reveals the many faces of the music-hall performer, stripping away the glamour of celebrity to unearth the imperfect human beings looming behind the grease paints and ostrich plumes.

Whereas makeup articulates exhaustion and fatigue in "The Halt," in "The Workroom" it connotes industry. Transporting readers backstage into a cramped, overheated, third-floor dressing room "saturated with the human odor of some sixty performers," the story follows five "girls" hastily preparing for their upcoming revue.[12] The only named character, a no-nonsense actor called Anita, moves quickly through the tiny space, pausing only to deftly uncover the feathered headdress featured in her next act. Desperate not to ruin the prop, Anita takes care because "everyone knows that grease powder, flying in clouds from shaken puffs, spells death to velvet and feathers" (117). As performers around her complain about the poor quality of their underclothes—abused from constant wear and paid for by the actors themselves out of their meager earnings—Anita chastises them for their incessant mewling. The pragmatic Anita abruptly turns "a half made-up face toward her companions, a dead-white mask with bright red goggles, that makes her look like a Polynesian warrior, and without even interrupting her tirade, she ties around her head a filthy rag, all that remains of a 'wig-kerchief,' intended to protect the hair from the brilliantine on the stage wigs" (118). Cosmetics thus not only animate the passionate Anita, bringing color and fire to her character; they also symbolize the performer's precarious economic status. Although they vehemently vocalize their discontent with theater practices and policies, especially those that they deem acutely unfair, Anita and the others are nevertheless careful not to spill grease powder because doing so would damage the expensive costumes that they can barely afford to purchase in the first place. Whereas Zola depicted the actor's loge as a site of male fantasy and portrayed the cosmetics within it as tools of erotic titillation, Colette provided a decidedly unromantic vision of both. In the cramped workspace of the loge, makeup was not presented as marking the bodies of sexually alluring performers but, rather, was matter-of-factly portrayed as a practical tool of the performer's trade.

In "Matinee," cosmetics illuminate the physical hardships engendered by the unrelenting pace of music-hall work as well as the performer's frustrations with the demands of her profession. Although the story depicts a pause, a moment when the mime is backstage between back-to-back revues, there is no sense of tranquility, no sense that the intermission is at all a break. At her dressing table, the overheated, worn-out performer finds that her "cold cream is unrecognizable, reduced to a cloudy oil that smells of gasoline. A melted paste, the color of rancid butter, is all that remains of my white grease foundation. The liquefied contents of my rouge jar might well be used to 'color,' as cooks say, a dish of *pêches Cardinal.*"[13] Wilted, melted, and soured—the rouge, the cold cream, and foundations remind the performer of herself. Like her, they have lost their luster, their freshness, and their ability to express beauty.

Despite her distaste for these overworked tools, the actress applies them dutifully, resigned that "for better or worse, here I am anointed with these multi-colored fats and heavily powdered" (121). Unwilling to completely forfeit the game, the mime, Colette explains, attempts to "survey a face on which glow, in the sunshine, the mixed hues of purple petunia, begonia, and the afternoon of blue morning glory" (121). Successful at refreshing her makeup and, by extension, bringing her own actor's face back to life, the performer nevertheless confesses her limitations: "But the energy to move, walk, dance, and mime, where can I hope to find that?" (121). Makeup enables the actress to look the part, but it fails to afford her either the strength or the endurance to perform her role.

Chronicling a moment in the life of a young dancer, "Love" showcases makeup's capacity to simultaneously distinguish and homogenize its wearers. Intrigued by Gloria, the most recent addition to the troupe, the narrator explains that "when she emerges from the dressing room she shares with her companions next to mine, and walks down towards the stage, ready made-up and in costume, I can't distinguish her from the other girls, for she strives, as is most fitting, to be just an impersonal and attractive little English dancer in a revue!"[14] Sporting matching costumes and faces painted to similar effect, the dancers lose all individuality, blurring seamlessly one into the other. "The nine faces are painted with identical makeup, cleverly tinted with mauve around the eyes, while the lids are burdened, on each of their lashes, with such a heavy touch of mascara that it is impossible to distinguish the true color of the pupil" (126). Colette's precise language here—eye lids "cleverly tinted" and lashes "burdened" by the "heavy touch of mascara"—reveals the effort required to craft a convincing artist's mask. Creating the illusion of uniformity, portraying the generic character of the "impersonal and attractive" chorus girl, demands that each dancer sublimate her personal identity to the persona that she will embody on stage. That Gloria, the newest member of the entourage, manages to already have learned this so well speaks to the performer's ability to relinquish herself entirely to her craft.

Onstage, Gloria effectively conforms to the standards of chorus-line appearance; however, backstage (and out of character) she garners the attention not only of the narrator but also of her fellow troubadour, the jack-of-all-trades Marcel. Infatuated, Marcel openly pursues Gloria—waiting for her after shows, sharing sweets, and attempting to engage her in conversation despite a significant language barrier. Unversed in the cultural cues embedded in her suitor's flirtations, Gloria fails to encourage Marcel's pursuit. Convinced that she is not interested in him, Marcel abandons the chase, leaving the confused Gloria brokenhearted. Witness to the debacle, the narrator characterizes it bluntly as nothing more than a commonplace consequence of life on the road. Nomadic by nature, performers quickly lose interest in that which they cannot attain and eagerly move on to the next conquest. Comparing traveling showgirls to gypsies ready to abandon their post, the narrator uses the showgirl's makeup cabinet as evidence of the performer's necessarily transient existence. In the cabinet, "red and black cosmetic pencils roll all over the makeup table, covered at one end with brown paper and at the other with a tattered towel. . . . The jar of rouge, the Leichner eyebrow pencil, the woolen powder puff, could all be carried away in a knotted handkerchief" (127). Ready to move at a moment's notice, the tools of the professional's trade—the rouge, the eyebrow pencil, the woolen powder puff—are as likely to be "carried away in a knotted handkerchief" as Gloria is to be replaced by another lover or even by another "little dancer."

Colette's short stories strip away the glitz and glamour patrons associated with the Belle Époque music hall to expose the harsh realities of life behind the scenes. Indeed, Colette so greatly admired and respected the people behind the spectacle that she did all she could to publicly legitimize stage work. Not only was the work itself demanding, but the "artists," she believed, "did not have time for fake personalities [offstage]; they were unadulterated human beings."[15] The scholar Patricia Tilburg argues that Colette embraced "an uncommon notion of the performer,"[16] one that united wage-paying manual labor with domestic order. Tilburg attributes this association to Colette's personal experiences within France's school system. Republican pedagogues promoted the cultivation of one's interior life through a variety of activities, regular physical labor chief among them. By focusing on the performer as a laborer rather than as celebrity, Colette portrayed "performance as craft" and situated music-hall work "within a long, honorable tradition of artisanal pride."[17]

Importantly, it was through the prism of stage makeup that Colette elected to illuminate how performers navigated the ubiquitous tension between beauty and work that defined all aspects of the music-hall experience. Performers worked hard to appear beautiful onstage; however, they intentionally hid their labors from the spectators for whom they toiled in order to make the stage performance appear both beautiful and effortless. Constantly becoming and unbecoming characters, accommodating and sublimating the "scattered selves" as they emerged through work and play, Colette's performers were caught in a state of perpetual transformation. Makeup played a privileged role in this process, paradoxically revealing that which it was intended to conceal.[18] For Colette, makeup did not merely enliven the stage siren or superficially embellish the already pretty face of a charming chanteuse; rather, it articulated the fragility and grit characteristic of the hardworking performers without whom the music hall itself could not survive.

BEAUTY IN THE PRESS: PRODUCING THE EVERYDAY

Colette's music-hall stories for *Le matin* comprised only a small percentage of her overall submissions to the periodical press. In fact, Colette's contribution to France's flourishing early-twentieth-century print culture was both extensive and varied. Scholars estimate that, by age seventy, Colette had authored more than 1,260 press articles.[19] Before making her literary début with the

Claudine series, she wrote music criticism for Maurice Barrès's short-lived review *La cocarde* in the 1890s. It was from these articles that Willy discovered and encouraged his wife's literary talent. Her next engagement with the press, which involved the serialization of Claudine under her husband's name, marked the beginning of the lifelong relationship that Colette would cultivate between her fiction and periodical print culture.

Between the 1890s and the 1950s, the press serialized dozens of Colette's novels, but her early forays into periodical writing also shaped her journalistic career. Ever the dedicated student, Colette used these early occasions to learn how to work under deadline and to meet the demands of a mass readership. In the 1910s, she serialized works in the popular magazine *La vie parisienne;* in the 1920s she wrote short stories for *Le Journal;* and in the 1920s and 1930s, she published frequently in the celebrity magazines *Gil Blas* and *Fantasio* and provided two weekly columns to the dailies *Le journal* and *Paris soir.*[20]

The press not only provided Colette with an important venue to showcase her fictive works, but it also offered her a public, commercial venue for trying her hand at nonfiction. Colette authored countless essays, news articles, and theatrical and literary reviews. She proved herself an able and intrepid reporter, tackling topics as controversial as domestic violence and the plight of the unemployed, and she became one of the first women to report from the front during the Great War. In 1910, she signed on with *Le matin,* the French daily with the second-largest circulation in Europe, to write a regular semimonthly column for the literary page, "Contes des mille et un matins." One staff journalist balked at the hire, refusing to work with "that circus performer," and an editor threatened to resign. The newspaper's managers feared that Colette's reputation might offend subscribers, and, under their guidance, Colette agreed initially to suppress her identity by writing under a pseudonym.[21] Within two months of her inaugural contribution, however, public interest in the mysterious author grew to such a fever pitch that Colette ended her January 27 installment with the coy confession, "It's me, Colette Willy."[22]

In addition to her critical reviews and serialized fiction, Colette penned dozens of pieces devoted to fashion, love, food, gardening, motherhood, physical culture, and beauty. She enthusiastically instructed women in how to care for their homes, families, and bodies. Mainstream dailies like *Le matin* and *Demain* routinely included articles in which Colette critiqued the latest fashions or championed a new beauty trend. Meanwhile, frequent contributions to magazines like *Femina* and *Vogue,* then later *Votre beauté* and *Marie-*

Claire, solidified Colette's reputation as a "woman's writer." In the press, Colette posed as a personal counselor, confidante, matriarch, and friend. But her writings also enabled her to make beauty a matter of public discourse and, in so doing, to acknowledge the hard work involved in creating oneself as nothing but a woman.

Many of Colette's contributions charmed readers with witty satires rooted in the experiences of everyday life. For example, in "Make-up," a short essay published in *Demain* in June 1924, Colette hyperbolized the average woman's overly complicated toilette. The narrator, Colette, encounters a male friend, "Z," at a perfumer's shop and is surprised to find him inspecting lipstick and rouge. When the saleswoman denies his request to try out the products, he agrees to purchase them all. "Five or six cylinders of gilt metal and a minute phial were handed over to my friend," Colette reports. "Very seriously and with a cynicism I found disconcerting[, he was] painting his lips conscientiously."[23] Baffled by this unusual act, Colette exclaims, "You're hideous! . . . have you gone mad?" Despite her outcry, Z persists in his experiment, applying one lipstick after the other before moving on to the rouge.

After selecting his favorites, he proclaims that his wife "will be delighted," to which the narrator replies, "They're for her?" (71). "No, my dear," he retorts, "They're for me. This make-up that turns my wife's mouth pimento-red, strawberry, tomato, delights the eyes. . . . But it's I who eat them" (71). Z patiently explains that he is madly in love with his wife but that every time he kisses her, his affections are met with putrid paints and foul-tasting artificial infusions. In an effort to prevent such distasteful encounters, Z has started choosing the products that his wife will wear. Amused by this odd arrangement, Colette asks if he ever sees his wife "properly washed," to which Z replies: "Washed! That's not the half of it! Scrubbed, polished, scraped with an ivory spatula, rubbed with an ether swab and boiling water, finally carefully coated with a camphor pomade to prevent wrinkles" (72). Despite herself, Colette cannot help but offer her own advice for the wife's toilette: "Start Marcelle off again on the glycerine cream, which I recall as sugary, even a little vanilla-flavored." As they approach Z's home, the conversation trails off, Z warning Colette that "My wife gets up late, we'll catch her at her toilette. I'm afraid of what may have happened in my absence" (72). Indeed, Colette discloses, "he had good reason to fear," for when they happen upon Marcelle, her face is covered in the "dregs of a cesspit," and she is unceremoniously scolding her little dog who has had the audacity to have been caught "rolling in something dirty!" (72).

Beneath the valance of humor and irony, Colette's story advances a poignant, if subtle, cultural commentary. Cleverly subverting social norms and conflating the serious with the trivial, Colette uses the medium of makeup to illustrate how gender roles are negotiated through everyday practices. Premised on an outlandish inversion—a man selecting, wearing, and purchasing beauty products—the story challenges assumptions about the role makeup plays in the lives of both men and women. Although it is the wife who, as would be expected, wears the makeup, it is the husband who is destined to "eat" it. Makeup, in this context, is not a feminine frivolity but a potentially dangerous weapon threatening to disrupt conjugal happiness. As a remedy to this clear and present danger, the husband vets products rather than discourage his wife from using them altogether. Certainly, he appreciates the visual effects that cosmetics elicit, but he also understands that, despite his aversion, his wife will not forego her beauty routine. Embedded in this refusal is the provocative suggestion that Marcelle beautifies not for her husband but for herself. By closing the story with the wife's condemnation of the family dog for "rolling in something dirty," a crime of which she herself is guilty, Colette suggests that while the use of artifice should be accepted as a serious component of feminine self-production, one need not ignore its playful aspects.

Colette reiterates makeup's centrality to everyday life in the multiple meanings she ascribes to the title itself. In the story, "makeup" carries several connotations concurrently. At the most basic level, the title indicates that the story is about makeup—cosmetic products that reside at the center of the narrative. But makeup also mediates the relationship between Z and Marcelle: it is Z's distaste for Marcelle's makeup that causes tension within the couple; it is Z's decision to choose cosmetics for his wife that comes to define their conjugal roles; it is this arrangement that mends the couple's bond and that covers over past disputes; and finally, it is this agreement that enables the couple to literally make up, to reconcile their differences and reestablish harmony in their home.

Colette returned to the theme of beautification as central to woman's self-production in her contributions to *Femina*. Featuring news from high society alongside articles documenting current events, women's forays into the workforce, and their participation in athletics, *Femina* also devoted countless pages to the adornment of domestic interiors and of female bodies. Sumptuously illustrated and widely read, *Femina* appealed to readers' lifestyle fantasies by offering a visually rich, if admittedly upper-middle-class "catalogue of modern femininity."[24] Although *Femina* advanced its own idealized vision of modern womanhood, the journal neither endeavored to unilaterally dictate its agenda nor to uncompromisingly impart its values to impressionable readers. Assiduously attentive to reader concerns and responsive to real changes under way in French politics and society, *Femina* adapted to the times and asked its readers to do the same.[25]

Lenard Berlanstein argues that in its first decade of publication, *Femina,* under the leadership of the publisher Pierre Lafitte, envisioned a "modern femininity" in which women's empowerment presented itself "as a practical necessity rather than an ideological imperative."[26] Pointing to Lafitte's establishment of prizes for women's artistic and literary works in 1903 and his prize for female aviators in 1910, Berlanstein contends that despite *Femina*'s initial antisuffragist stance (which it revised in 1909 in accordance with reader attitudes), the journal unequivocally supported woman's sociopolitical advancement.[27] The journal was careful to communicate, however, that in encouraging women to pursue a wide range of activities outside the home, it did not advocate a masculinization of women themselves; in fact, the magazine went out of its way to show how women could, by harnessing their charm, elegance, and seductiveness, achieve their goals without losing their femininity.[28]

Despite its attentiveness to the glamorous "good life," *Femina* continued to address more practical reader concerns and to welcome feedback. In its June 1920 issue, for example, *Femina* offered a petite "Livre de madame," a concise beauty advice column (it included eight paragraphs on makeup application and a few comments on maintaining the mouth and combating wrinkles) intended to rival the more elaborate beauty manuals that overflowed unnecessarily with "*grand mots*" and that more often than not endorsed only expensive products.[29] The magazine also maintained its well-established practice of surveying subscribers.[30] A few months before publishing "Le livre de madame," the contributor Claire Launay asked readers, "Pour qui une femme s'habille t'elle?" Launay proposed three options: "for men," "for other women," or "for oneself." While many respondents selected one of the proffered choices, others wrote in "for the world" or "for one's age." Adapting to the interests of its readers, *Femina* not only acknowledged the write-in options but also published responses submitted in all five categories. By identifying respondents as "madam," "mademoiselle," "a patricienne," "Baronne," and a "celibataire de 21 ans," the magazine also revealed the range in social class, age, and marital status of its readers.[31]

In her columns on the subject for *Femina,* Colette presented rituals of beautification as important feminine rites of passage. Portraying herself as a beauty expert, Colette advised readers on the best skin-care products and the most effective techniques for applying makeup. She also led by example; for instance, when she praised Defossée's perm as a "brilliant invention," she modeled it herself, keeping her hair permed and dyed mauve for the next thirty years. To convey her expertise, her articles often took on a maternal tone. Playing the role of doting mother in a 1927 article for *Femina* entitled "Fards, poudres, parfums," Colette disguised her advice as a letter to and about her daughter. Importantly, Colette's article appreciated the complexity of the beauty ritual at a historical moment when feminine dress was becoming increasingly simplified. Cosmetics, as Colette portrayed them, enabled women to distinguish themselves and to experiment with their "look" even as sartorial trends became more undifferentiated and uniform. She described her fifteen-year-old daughter's fascination with makeup, the new "jouets de femmes," and confided to readers explicitly how Bel-Gazou had been seduced by the array of colors and types of products available. She condoned the young girl's obsession with her appearance, arguing that makeup had become "inoffensive" in the 1920s and as "ordinary as food."[32] She not only normalized these once-transgressive beauty aids, but she celebrated them as markers of feminine maturity: "What is important is that my daughter plays. She approaches her satin temple with shades of coral, clear, and medium; she hesitates, clamps her mouth, bursts with laughter. Her face is still child-like, but on it is the mask of the future wife." Comparing various Lucien Lelong products to ripe fruits and flowers, she encouraged her daughter to "poudre-toi!" to celebrate her youth, and to discover her individuality.[33] In short, by offering advice about cosmetics and by sharing the secrets of self-performance, Colette welcomed her offspring (and her readers) into womanhood.

Colette revisited these themes in her contributions to *Vogue.* In addition to focusing on the season's latest fashion trends and reporting on the personal lives of cosmopolitan socialites, *Vogue* devoted a good deal of copy to rituals of beautification.[34] Indeed, the number of *Vogue* articles about cosmetics and other beauty aids grew steadily during its first decade of publication in France. In 1920, for example, articles like "Charm and Grace" and "Men's Attitudes about Women's Fashions" reflected the magazine's concentration on issues of comportment and fashion.[35] By 1929, articles such as "Makeup for Evening," which explained how to use color to harmonize the eye with artificial light, and "Beauty Products," which highlighted a handful of useful creams, serums, and powders for the transition from summer to autumn, exemplified *Vogue*'s sustained interest in beauty culture.[36]

Vogue's support was further evidenced in its inclusion of countless advertisements for health and beauty aids. Firms took out full-page ads for cosmetics, hair products, skin creams, aesthetic treatments, and institutes. Certainly, *Vogue* benefitted financially from this arrangement. In 1924, firms paid upward of five thousand francs for a one-page ad—a price that increased to seven thousand francs by 1934.[37] Despite the high price of placing an ad, the number of advertisements for beauty products (excluding perfumes) and beauty institutes grew throughout the 1920s (see table 4.1). Although the number of ads fell somewhat dramatically through the 1930s, likely in response to the economic crisis of those years, they nevertheless remained vibrant and never fell lower than the number placed in the first year of the magazine's run in France.[38]

Lengthy articles, like one from March 1921 entitled, "La philosophie de la poudre et du fard," exemplified *Vogue's* recognition that beautification was at the top of woman's agenda. The unidentified author opened with a play on a line from Victor Hugo's 1828 poem "L'enfant," which commemorated the Greek War of Independence. Hugo's abandoned child confides to the narrator

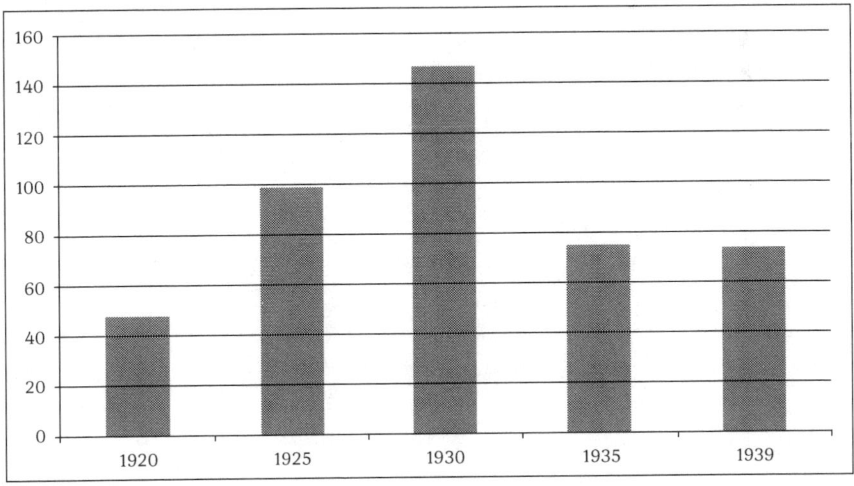

Table 4.1. Number of Beauty Product and Institute Advertisements in *Vogue*, 1920–1939.

after the massacre at Chios, "I want powder and bullets." Today's child, however, the *Vogue* writer contends, prefers "powder and blush."[39] The implication here is that the battle cry of today's young person is not for weapons of violence, but for weapons of beauty. A new war for independence is raging, and to fight the good fight a young woman needs both powder and blush. From here, the author boldly champions "Powder, the symbol of liberty!" and moves on to a discussion of aesthetic currents and woman's efforts to reproduce herself as a work of art. Cautioning against the abuse of cosmetics and the overapplication of color, the writer explains that beautification "demands infinite delicacy [and] measure, if not science."[40] Women need appreciate, moreover, that "it is as great an art to make up as it is a great art to paint; a grave error consists when one imagines grabbing a powder puff, a pencil or applicator, and expects to transform the face instantly."[41] Thus women need not only be equipped with the weapons of warfare, they must also be skilled in the tactics of combat.

Vogue contributors echoed the sentiments of the author quoted above and encouraged women to use products efficaciously and to good effect. In "De l'importance d'être belle," one *Vogue* contributor explained: "The form and proportion of the face and its traits, the color of the skin, the personality, the hour of day, the color of the outfit, all of this must be taken into account."[42] This author went on to suggest that every woman should purchase superior products and know the quality of her face (oily or dry skin) before applying the correct product for the time of day.[43] Contributors encouraged women to seek counsel in institutes, to learn how to match their makeup with their complexions, their lifestyles, the occasion, and even the time of day; and they urged women to "take advantage of all of the tools available." In her article "Quelques secrets sur l'art d'être belle," Mme. M. T. Sylviac, for example, advocated "rigorous" hygiene (cleansing, toning, moisturizing), dividing the face into symmetrical sections in order to administer to each feature, and even consulting a physician.[44] The magazine was so invested in teaching women appropriate application procedures that, in 1931, it teamed with Elizabeth Arden and the Worth fashion house to create makeup lines that harmonized each year's fashionable colors with women's skin types, ages, hair colors, and activities.[45]

A frequent contributor to *Vogue* throughout the 1920s, Colette engaged a variety of topics related to the intimate issues of a woman's daily life. From "Holidays" to "Hats," "Visits" to "Captive Gardens," Colette's eloquent, often evocative essays elevated the routine aspects of woman's quotidian life, rendering them worthy of comment and deserving of appreciation. In satirical lighthearted stories, "Tomorrow's Springtime," "Models," and "Elegance, Economy" (all of which appeared in *Vogue* in 1925), Colette employed her characteristic wit to expose the effort and anxiety involved in creating and performing the ordinary female self.

The narrator in "Tomorrow's Springtime" woefully anticipates the next season's fashions. While vacationing in Nice, she notices the ridiculously short, appallingly tight skirts adopted by the fashionable set about town. Certain that these trends will dominate the spring lines in Paris, she laments that 1925 will be "fatal again for those women whom Nature has provided with unambiguous contours. It is true that the species is becoming rare."[46] Disgusted by the flat, short skirts that strip women of their curves, turning them into nothing more than "slim lamp post[s]," Colette challenges both the aesthetics and the practicality of the look. For when these lamp posts sit down, she points out, "their short, tight, sweet, miserable little skirts will ride up beyond what is permissible, exposing stockings to which inflexible whim has given the exact shade of the dolls we used to make out of bran" (34–35). Transformed into uncomfortable rag dolls, women who follow the new fashions participate in their own subjugation. However, they are only partly to blame because it is not the female wearer but the male couturier who is guilty of creating restrictive women's clothing without asking "you for your opinion" (35). Colette's concern here is thus not woman's desire to appear attractive or fashionable but with the designers whose clothing protracts woman's freedom of movement and hides her feminine curves. In effect, Colette exposes the gap between the imagined woman, the waif-like lamp post envisioned by the male couturier, and the real woman, the woman with flesh and breasts condemned to wear fashions that limit her mobility and mask her femininity.

Colette again explores the relationship between real and imagined women in "Models." Watching the men who accompany their wives to Paris's fashion shows, the narrator claims, "only men derive a total pleasure, unmarred by covetousness, from the parade of models."[47] Men enjoy this privilege not merely because they like to admire the figures of pretty girls, but because, unlike their female counterparts, they do not attempt to envision their own bodies adorned in the fashions on display. The narrator describes women in the audience as "secretly frantic" as they "broken-heartedly" renounce "a little 'creation' at six thousand francs"; meanwhile, "the man beams, observes, takes note of X's low waistline and Z's draperies as he might absorb the characteristic of a school of painting" (39). This detachment, moreover, enables man to "appreciate the *ensemble* better than the woman. He can assess the model quite objectively, better than the woman" (39). The main difference between husband and wife is the husband's recognition that the clothing he admires was made to be worn not by his wife (a real woman) but by a model (an imagined woman).

Fascinated by the role that the model herself plays in this illusion, the narrator identifies her as a "disturbing colleague," an "end point of a concerted effort that everyone now recognizes" (39). Like the men in the audience, the narrator also distances herself from the model; however, rather than view the model as the ideal woman, she regards her as a sexless, disembodied inanimate object—a culmination, an "end point." "The public appreciates the part played by the weaver, the designer, the cutter, the saleswoman, the couturier who directs them all; but, as far as the model is concerned, it is more reserved, it ponders—admiring or suspicious" (40). Although implicated in the creative process and associated with the chain of production (the weaver, the cutter, the designer, the saleswoman), the model as product contributes to her (or, in the narrator's words, "its") own commodification. "Among all the modernized aspects of the most luxurious industries, the model, a vestige of voluptuous barbarism, is like some plunder-laden prey. She is the object of unbridled regard, a living bait, the passive realization of an ideal" (40). She is, in her objectified state, a combination of the real and the imagined woman, but by playing at both, she successfully embodies neither.

The model's liminal positioning in the social and sexual order is reinforced by her moral ambiguity. "No other female occupation contains such potent impulses to moral disintegration as this one," the narrator asserts, "applying as it does the outward signs of riches to a poor and beautiful girl" (40). Strange, capricious, the model moves fluidly yet disconcertingly through society, disrupting the regulatory norms of sex, gender, and class as she personifies the latest trend. "Beauty," the narrator chides, "is meant for admiration and you [designer] fit her out to increase this admiration" (40). Casting her to embody an ideal, the designer reinforces the model's precarious social station and contributes to the erasure of her humanity. Implicit in the narrator's critique is not only that this arrangement disadvantages models but also that it threatens the real women who endeavor to look like her—to wear the fashions at six thousand francs. By idolizing the empty model, the average woman risks losing sight of the real—a disconnect that could alienate her from both the ideal she reveres and the genuine self she sacrifices in its pursuit.

Colette demonstrates how fashion structures the ordinary woman's everyday life in a third essay, "Elegance, Economy." The narrator recounts a series of encounters with her friend Valentine, a practical Parisian whose budget prohibits her from affording the "thirty-six outfits" necessary to accommodate every change of weather. Uncertain how Valentine derived at thirty-six as the suitable number of outfits for the average woman, the narrator insists "on knowing whether, in a feminine budget, economy need banish elegance, that supreme elegance that consists of wearing the right garment at the right time, in the right place and circumstances."[48] Half-serious, half-mocking, the narrator's inquiry illustrates how hard the average woman must work to meet the sartorial norms governing female comportment. A woman prepared for an emergency, Valentine's pragmatic approach to self-fashioning leads her to pursue only the most functional trends, notably the adoption of the bob hairstyle. "When she had her hair cut short she thought she'd wake up in the morning with her hair done once and for all. But the coiffeur, lord of the curls, pruner of the neck, with the copyright of a certain twist of hair by the ear, was alert; and I know many a freed woman who already groans: 'Oh, it's too much . . . I shall have to cut it every fortnight'" (43). Pointing out the irony behind the hairstyle intended to liberate and touted for its ease of care, Colette playfully teases the women whom "laziness" has distracted from "healthy and vigilant coquetry" (43).

After poking fun at the shrewd Valentine, the narrator generalizes her critique, asking: "Decked out and groomed at ten o'clock like prize horses, how many women approach their second toilette with any eagerness? How many of you are nonchalantly content with a 'paint-job' performed in a restaurant cloakroom? Powder and rouge in clouds, a stroke of the comb, a brushing of hands and nails . . ."? (43). Exposing "healthy and vigilant coquetry" as a series of quickie paint jobs clandestinely carried out in restaurant cloakrooms, Colette mocks the clouds of powder and rouge that enable women to deck themselves out like "prize horses." By poking fun at both the practical Valentine and the dedicated woman of fashion who carries out her second toilette despite her lack of eagerness for it, Colette reveals coquetry as an almost absurd, time-consuming labor. Her point here is not that women should forego self-care but rather that they should not allow it to rule their lives; they should strive to produce elegance economically.

In these essays from *Demain, Femina,* and *Vogue,* Colette used trivial commodities—makeup and fashion—to advance pointed social commentaries. Through humor and hyperbole, Colette tackled the delicate issue of power negotiation between a young husband and wife in "Make-up." Sensitive to what Z perceives as his wife's silly obsession, Colette adroitly illustrates how woman's pursuit of her own desires (in this case the desire to beautify) threatens conjugal harmony. Rather than dissuade Z from his efforts or chastise Marcelle for her habits, Colette advises the pair on products upon which they might both agree. In so doing, she subtly condones the wife's activities and indicates her approval of the husband's willingness to do the same. Playing the role of confidante in "Fards, poudres, parfums," Colette depicts the use of makeup as a valuable rite of passage. By envisioning cosmetics as an essential tool of feminine self-creation, she implores readers to acknowledge woman's agency in her own making and to take beauty itself seriously. Finally, in the selections from *Vogue,* Colette challenges the fashion industry's capacity to constrain the female body. Rather than become slaves to fashion (and to fashion designers), Colette encourages women to actively participate in their own self-fashioning. Disguised as quaint tales about makeup and clothing, Colette's stories poignantly illuminate the complicated politics involved in the ordinary process of becoming a woman.

LIVING TO BE BEAUTIFUL: LA SOCIÉTÉ COLETTE

Throughout the first three decades of the twentieth century, Colette the music-hall performer, novelist, and journalist relied upon her svelte body and her ink pen to literally and figuratively bring beautiful women to life. In the summer of 1931, as France began to experience the effects of global economic depression, the indefatigable Colette took her academic interest in feminine beauty to the next level by launching her own *institut de beauté.* Thrilled by the prospect of "touching the living flesh, heightening its colors, concealing its defects with my impartial fingers," and "inspired by a kind of benevolent, maternal feeling," Colette enthusiastically embarked upon her new business venture. Undeterred by the country's perilous fiscal situation and unconcerned about the inevitable criticism of her peers, Colette submitted to her desire to "find the women beautiful as they emerge from beneath my writer's fingers."[49]

Introduced to Paris by Valentin Le Brun in 1895, exclusive beauty institutes gradually populated the capital city in the first decades of the twentieth century. At this time, celebrities and esteemed aestheticians brought the latest treatments, products, and techniques to an equally cosmopolitan clientele. The steady increase in the number of institutes before the war, however, paled in comparison to their meteoric growth after it.[50] As a *Beauté* magazine columnist reported in 1929, "The rise in the number of beauty institutes since the war is stunning."[51] Indeed, new institutes appeared regularly: Phébel and Elizabeth Arden (1920), Jeanne Gatineau (1922), Cédib (1924), and Payot (1925) provide but a few examples of this phenomenon. What was equally impressive to the journalist was that the institute's success was "not only a consequence of fashion" but also the result of an influx of trained aestheticians and cosmetologists, who provided sound advice about "effective, scientific application."[52] Institutes employed a variety of "specialists" (hairdressers, aestheticians, masseuses, even doctors and chemists) and provided a wide range of professional services (facials, manicures, weight-loss programs, and cosmetic surgery). The majority of salons, moreover, were launched and administered by female directors. When Colette opened the doors to her new enterprise, she was certainly in good company, but she was also up against some fierce competition.

Any financially secure, business-savvy woman might open an institute; however, because name recognition was crucial to a successful launch, many *directrices* were celebrities or women who themselves were revered as great beauties.[53] In 1914, "opera's greatest beauty," Lina Cavalieri, retired from the stage to pursue two new passions: the cinema and the beauty profession.[54] At age forty, the celebrated chanteuse opened an institute featuring her own product line and skin-care systems not in Milan or Rome but at 61 avenue Victor-Emmanuel in Paris. In her institute, she sought to adapt routines "to the personality of each woman."[55] Portrayed in firm advertisements as "the grande artiste," Cavalieri created lipsticks and rouges composed of the most "active" ingredients and providing the most "intense" color. In addition to cosmetic products defined by their vibrancy, she offered protective skin-care systems that safely nourished the skin. Behind advertisements that emphasized the scientifically tested ingredients used to fabricate the firm's products and that extolled the latest application methods employed in its institutes was the implied promise that women who purchased these products or who followed her advice might learn how to look like Cavalieri herself. By featuring the singer prominently in its advertisements and conflating her products with her celebrity, the firm played on the ordinary woman's fantasies of extraordinary beauty and glamour.

The same year that Cavalieri opened her institute, she also contributed an advice column for *Femina* and published a book entitled *My Secrets of Beauty*. The publisher's foreword to the guide proclaimed that the "woman who owns this book will be freed forever from dependence upon unreliable 'beauty doctors' and expensive cosmetics of doubtful value."[56] Cavalieri's manual endorsed bathing practices, physical fitness and hygiene, remedies for skin maladies, and (unfortunately) the frequent use of gasoline shampoo! She interspersed her text with personal photos and images of beautiful celebrities, primarily from the opera, who defined for her the current beauty standard. "The beautiful woman has points," she wrote. "Let us enumerate them: A figure graceful in outline, not too thin, nor too fat. A face that is fascinating and by fascinating I mean interesting. But to make it interesting it must have what? Features that are well proportioned, let us say regular. They must also seem to belong to one's own face and no other." And, finally, the "nose must not be too large nor too small, but just large enough for the face in which it is set."[57] Cavalieri's perceptive decision to publish her manual and her column concurrently with the launch of her institute demonstrated her business acumen at the same time that it announced the singer's foray into the beauty profession.

Cavalieri and other celebrities cum *directrices* had both flourishing business models and formidable competitors in two world-renowned beauty professionals, Helena Rubinstein and Elizabeth Arden. Rubinstein's success began in Australia, where she invented a cold cream with family member and Hungarian chemist Jacob Lykusky. Working with Lykusky, Rubinstein developed what would become the three signature components of her wildly successful skin-care regime: cold cream to cleanse, astringent to close pores, and vanishing cream to moisturize and protect.[58] She opened a small shop in Melbourne, where her creams became all the rage among the city's most fashionable women. In response to this popularity, Rubinstein began manufacturing larger quantities of product, and she started to diversify her line. Shortly thereafter, she launched a salon in London, and then, in 1912, she opened shop in Paris. Following a different path, Florence Nightingale Graham started out as a low-paid "treatment girl" in Eleanor Adair's salon before joining the cosmetologist Elizabeth Hubbard in her New York institute. Once Graham developed her own line of products, she opened her first institute in New York City under the name Elizabeth Arden. Although it was 1920 before Arden launched her Paris institute, she, like Rubinstein, would enjoy tremendous success selling her skin-care systems and beautification methods to French consumers.

Launching institutes and distribution sites across the globe, Rubinstein and Arden attempted to move beyond the storefront to secure diverse markets for their products. Both women incorporated manufacturing units within their companies (Rubinstein in 1917, Arden in 1918), and both sought high-volume product sales.[59] In response to demand for her "pasteurized" creams, Rubinstein opened a small manufacturing outlet in St. Cloud that employed twenty-five workers in bottling and labeling.[60] In 1923, Arden dispatched her relative Gladys Graham to Paris to supervise her expanding operations there, which included wholesale and manufacturing divisions. The Arden institute relocated a year later to 2 rue de la Paix because it had grown too large for its original building.[61] Although Rubinstein and Arden did not begin their empires in Paris (in fact, it is likely that they established manufacturing centers there because of the high taxes on imports and exports imposed in postwar France), once established in the city, they thrived.[62] Advertising their expensive treatment lines in high-end magazines like *Vogue* and selling them in their institutes and in the elite shops of Paris, Rubinstein and Arden successfully infiltrated the competitive French cosmetics market.[63]

Encouraged by these female entrepreneurs, Colette, who entertained a lifelong obsession with creams and paints, envisioned a beauty business of her own. Colette's mother (Sido) taught her when she was a very young girl to condition and style her long, shiny plaited hair with concoctions made from herbs in the family garden. Meanwhile, in primary school she learned the values of *morale laïque*—a republican philosophy that regarded the body as an instrument of moral improvement. As she matured, Colette valued a body that was morally disciplined and physically conditioned. Cleanliness and good personal hygiene were essential to achieving this ideal body. Even during her many years on stage, as she learned to use paints and kohls to dramatic effect, Colette never promoted artifice as a wholly satisfactory substitute for a well-made body. But the body could use help, and by the time she opened her institute, at the apex of her celebrity, she had undergone a rudimentary facelift, cosmetic dental work, and several experimental hair surgeries!

A devoted physical culturalist from a young age, Colette graced the November 15, 1911, cover of the bimonthly *La culture physique*. The cover featured

Colette's toned body draped in a bed sheet and included the simple headline "Colette Willy: Fervent Fan of Physical Culture," a possible double entendre for Colette's adoration for both exercise and the magazine that promoted it.[64] Colette maintained her obsession with bodily care throughout her life. Jacques Gauither-Villars recalls his stepmother primping in the bathroom for at least an hour every morning, and he notes that she often mixed her own beauty aids in the kitchen sink.[65] In fact, Colette had dabbled briefly in the cosmetics industry before the war, when, under Willy's direction, she authorized the sale of a line of Claudine powders (along with a variety of other novelties) to promote her novels by the same name.

In 1931, Colette finally made cosmetics a priority, and she devoted herself wholeheartedly to the success of her new business. Before she could break ground on her project, however, she needed to secure financial support. Assisted by her third husband, Maurice Goudeket, she courted investors, including the Pasha of Marrakech and the Princesse de Polignac, who along with three other backers provided 1 million francs in start-up funds.[66] When the company was incorporated as La Société Colette for the manufacture of beauty products in March 1932, Colette not only lent her name to her product line but also committed countless hours to establishing a product research laboratory and to personally developing compound formulae. She reported to her friend Hélène Picard in November 1931 that she had created one perfume and two tonics for different skin types, but that she was behind in her development of lipsticks and creams. When not occupied in the laboratory, Colette busied herself creating packaging for her products, producing flyer advertisements, and hand-drawing her own portrait on the boxes of powder that would occupy the shelves of her outlets.

Given her attention to the fabrication, packaging, and advertising of her products, it is not surprising that when the partners found a site for the institute in Paris's fashionable eighth arrondissement, Colette herself supervised the renovation of the building's interior. Everything about the look of the institute was modern: its art deco design, its mirrored walls, its chrome-accented leather armchairs, its glass-and-nickel countertops, its white shelves displaying little black pots bearing Colette's signature and profile, and even its staff adorned in crisp white lab coats. Colette personally wrote out the invitations announcing the institute's grand opening: "I inaugurate my beauty products boutique Wednesday, June 1—I will be happy, Madame, to welcome you myself, 6 rue de Miromesnil, and guide you in your choice of the most becoming makeup for the stage, or for the town."[67] And, despite illness and fatigue, Colette, sporting a crisp, no-nonsense black-and-white suit, eagerly greeted each inquisitive guest at the front door. Overcome with the excitement of it all, she gushed in another letter to Hélène: "The potential is very good. Curiosity takes care of us. And I'll send a small package, powder and cream. My shop would please you so much! It is very different from what I had imagined: I once thought it would be a kind of Batignolles grocery, with a tiled stove and a pot to cook the chestnuts, and the cat on the counter.... Alas, we must sacrifice to the taste of the age. But it is very gay, and very nice."[68] At age sixty, the esteemed author of the Claudine novels, *Chéri,* and *La vagabonde,* as well as dozens of novellas, essays, and press articles, traded her ink pen for an eyebrow pencil and tried her hand at the business of beauty.

Captivated by Colette's ostentatious undertaking, the press eagerly reported on the venture, inadvertently supplying the firm with (by Colette's account) fifty thousand francs in free publicity.[69] In the spring of 1932, the *Votre beauté* contributor Juliette Goublet interviewed the proud proprietor about her new endeavor.[70] Colette bragged to her star-struck interviewer that she designed the product packages herself and in her own image. In the design of her products, Colette could not resist the opportunity to once more play with her own subjectivity; inscribing product names onto her own recognizable profile, Colette blurred the line between her image and her products, offering herself as a commodity, an object for purchase. When asked what prompted her entrée into the manufacture of beauty aids, the vivacious entrepreneur immediately corrected: "Not start but continue.... I have always made my own cold cream.... I've been creating my own products for thirty-six years."[71] She then admitted that through the (sometimes reluctant) cooperation of friends and family members, she had learned how to make effective creams, powders, and liquid tonics. Having dispensed her advice and practiced her technique on a diverse population, Colette believed that she had created aids that could benefit all women, regardless of skin type or color. A labor of love, Colette considered her beauty work as more than a "little philanthropic." Comparing herself to a modern sorceress who passionately mixed products in her lab, Colette hoped that through her efforts, every woman might recapture her lost youth and reclaim "*de vraie vie.*"[72] For Colette, Goublet jubilantly ended her article, "to live and to be beautiful are the same thing."[73]

Despite Colette's enthusiasm for her new business, not everyone was as supportive of the scheme as the staff at *Votre beauté.* Critics alleged that by associating her name with a commercial enterprise, Colette valued revenue over reputation. Why would a revered member of the French literati willingly besmirch her good name by attaching it to a cosmetics line? Was it worth, they pressed, sullying the writer's image to hock something so mundane, so vulgar as a jar of rice powder? Many critics dismissed Colette's business as the latest episode in a long history of publicity-seeking escapades. Like the scandalous theatrical performances and racy prewar public appearances that preceded it, opening a beauty institute, critics charged, undermined her legitimacy as a woman of letters. These concerns undoubtedly provided an excuse for denying her the Legion d'honneur and for refusing her admission to L'Academie Goncourt, for both of which she was rumored to be under consideration in 1931. Convinced that the "circus performer" was at it again, critics relegated Colette to the margins of respectability even while she continued to win over the people of France, who overran her institutes, hoping to discuss the literature and to request the autograph (both of which Colette enthusiastically conceded) of one of France's greatest living authors.

Colette was well aware that her decision to peddle wrinkle creams and to perform facials could jeopardize her reputation; and yet she could not resist the opportunity to launch her own business, nor could she ignore her deep-seated desire to make women beautiful. Maurice claimed that Colette "always adored busying herself with the human face, she used to change the hair style of her friends, using the scissors for it, and even an unknown visitor would not be spared." She took great pleasure, he added, in "modifying faces, restoring their true characters to them, manipulating colours, plunging her hands deep into pastes and unguents."[74] According to Goudeket, Colette's interest in beauty work stemmed above all from its regenerative potential, what he called the "restoration of character." Colette derived infinite pleasure from watching, in awe, as women emerged beautiful "from beneath [her] writer's fingers." For Colette, the writing pen and the eyebrow pencil were not so very different.

Shortly after the doors opened to her Paris institute, in August 1931, Colette launched two product outlets, one in Saint-Tropez and another in Nantes. Over the course of the next year, she toured France exhibiting her products, offering beauty consultations, lecturing, and selling her cosmetics at provincial trade fairs and in Parisian department stores. Despite these efforts, Colette's business was in serious financial trouble by 1932. Exhausted, suffering through a series of health problems, and hemorrhaging capital, Colette reluctantly dissolved her beauty business in May 1933. By all accounts, she was better suited to writing about beauty than to actually making women beautiful.

Beauty aids were more than the props of femininity for Colette; they were agents of transformation. Colette believed that coloring one's hair, wearing grease paint and kohl, or experimenting with lipstick and powders provided women with new ways of becoming. As a beauty institute *directrice,* moreover, Colette encouraged women to cultivate artificial beauty and to regard such work not as a labor for others but as a rite of passage, a necessary diversion on the pathway to self-discovery. As such, cosmetics signified endless possibility: they allowed women to defy the "claw marks" of age, to armor against or to seduce the opposite sex, and to create themselves as both individuals and as women.

Announcing the first installment of Colette's serialized novel *La vagabonde,* the May 21, 1910, cover of the risqué weekly *La vie parisienne* featured a hypersexualized caricature of Renée Néré. Adorned in the gypsy's colorful, diaphanous fabrics, Renée, her back to the viewer, gazes intently into her dressing-table mirror to apply the grease paints for her next performance. Dark curly tendrils of hair, barely held in place by a cinched headscarf, frame her kohl-rimmed eyes and deep-red lips. Positioned as it is within a circle that mimics a telegraphic lens or a roughly hewn peephole, the image intentionally titillates. Metaphorically entrapped and visually captured in the viewer's voyeuristic gaze, the vagabond is caught in the act of producing the feminine.

How many times had Colette herself been ensnared in this same trap? Interrupted in the process of producing the feminine on stage, in her novels, or at home in front of her own looking glass? As a music-hall mime, a journalist assigned the task of assembling disparate snapshots of daily life, a cosmetics entrepreneur better suited to writing about beauty than to actually making women beautiful, Colette heroically confronted the gap between woman as individual and woman as image. For a woman who lived and worked in the public eye, Colette was acutely aware of the female body as an object perpetually on display. Her image might even be glimpsed in the picture of Renée—Renée tenuously holding herself together, representing the disjointed pieces of the author's usually scattered self. Colette—the author, the performer, the vagabond, the woman, the unadulterated human being—found expression not only through work but also through her work on beauty.

Makeup mattered for Colette. It mattered because as a conduit of self-fashioning, as a tool for self-creation, and as a strategy of self-presentation, it enabled woman to literally and metaphorically produce her self. Colette explored this phenomenon in each of her professional pursuits. In her music-hall essays, makeup marked the glamorous and the practical, it structured relationships, and it conveyed emotion. In her journalistic writings, makeup legitimized feminine beauty as a topic of public discourse and showed how everyday practices shaped social roles. And, in her business venture, Colette promoted makeup as a female passion and as a pathway to self-discovery. In every way for Colette, beauty marked the feminine, and makeup revealed the intimate; makeup was woman's most private secret, her lifelong profession, and her most trusted partner in the business of becoming nothing but a woman.

III
Modern Beauty

> Our time is a time of conspicuous colors and acute rhythms, of, if I dare say, aesthetic inflation. Woman wants to transcend. She wants to shine. Natural beauty, the rational maintenance of the body and the face is not enough! One needs a brighter glare, a mask that better accentuates the dynamic attractions suited to strike man's imagination with its first blow. The modern woman, above all, wants to be seen.
>
> —Dr. Nadia Grégoire Payot, *Être belle*

The distinguished hygienist and respected beauty advisor Dr. Nadia Grégoire Payot encouraged French women to use their beauty to make themselves visible within the vibrant landscape of the twentieth-century city. Amid boulevards punctuated by electric lamps, heaving with high-speed motorized vehicles, and teeming with bold placards, colorful signs, and illuminated storefronts, women increasingly competed for attention. Cautioning against merely blending into the spectacle, Payot persuaded women that "natural beauty, the rational maintenance of the body and the face is not enough!" All too aware of the challenges encountered when attempting to see and to be seen, the author implored women to cultivate a beauty that would enable them to "transcend" and to "shine." Encouraging women to pursue "a brighter glare" and to don "a mask that better accentuates the dynamic attractions suited to strike man's imagination with its first blow," Payot acknowledged woman's struggle to claim her place in the hectic postwar world.[1]

The Great War considerably facilitated woman's increased participation in public life. The wartime economy and the demand for women to replace men serving at the front in the workforce enabled many middle-class and working-class women to live independently. Working-class women left low-wage domestic service (especially after the unemployment benefit declined and the cost of living skyrocketed in 1916) for higher-paying jobs in the munitions, steel, and iron industries or to work in the service sector as public-transit operators, hairdressers, and salesclerks. As women entered into the university, the tertiary sector, and the factory as never before, familiar debates about woman's social role, her political relevance, and her ambiguous relationship to the opposite sex acquired a new salience.[2] Moreover, whereas their new women predecessors had appeared primarily in print media as caricatures and subjects of satire or were occasionally embodied by real-life figures like Colette, the women who emerged in the postwar decade constituted a pervasive mass phenomenon, infiltrating the streets of French cities large and small, moving freely in and out of mixed-class, heterosocial spaces, even emerging within the ranks of one's own family.[3]

Perhaps the single most unsettling type of modern woman to emerge in the postwar decade, the androgynous *garçonne* signified a complete break from women of the past. Youthful and assertive, the hedonistic *garçonne* served as a painful reminder of the war's upheaval at the same time that she rekindled debates about woman's social and political positions within the republic.[4] Noteworthy for her appearance—her bobbed hair, her adoption of masculine attire including trousers, ties, and even monocles—as well as for her unruly behavior (smoking, drinking, dancing shamelessly to jazz music), the *garçonne* threatened a status quo that desperately desired to return to prewar normalcy. Moreover, by creating herself in the image of man, the *garçonne,* critics alleged, abandoned her "true sex." In so doing, she not only trivialized the feminine but also undermined the conventions governing feminine beauty.

Yet the *garçonne*'s embrace of the masculine did not, as many contemporaries lamented, signify a total renunciation of the feminine. In her endeavor to create herself in the image of man, cultivating a boyish figure and cutting her hair, the *garçonne* relied heavily upon a range of *feminine* beauty practices, products, and services. Indeed, the *garçonne* was not a woman who had "lost her sex," as contemporary detractors alleged, but rather a woman who used conventionally feminine tools (fashion, cosmetics) to expose the arbitrariness of sex-based gender categories. Certainly, the *garçonne* mimicked male appearance in an effort to appropriate male power, but the play itself would not have been possible without the products and services that she accessed through France's feminine beauty culture. The great irony of the *garçonne,* then, was that in choosing to upset the gender order by comporting herself as a man, she relied on the very tools of femininity that had, for decades, distinguished her as a woman.

Understanding the *garçonne* in this way also suggests that, despite the social and economic opportunities engendered by the Great War, neither the *garçonne* nor modern womanhood generally should be understood simply as an inevitable by-product of the war experience. Indeed, Payot's declaration that modern women desired "to be seen," indicated the extent to which femininity was increasingly produced at the intersection of specific and intertwined commercial and cultural forces at work in the postwar period. For it was not only the greater presence of female bodies—on city streets, in places of business—but also the public display of those bodies in the media, in marketing materials, and on the stage that together influenced how French women were seen. Furthermore, the proliferation of female images generated multiple versions of womanhood that, though primarily metropolitan and middle-class, nevertheless conditioned ordinary women to see their selves and their bodies anew. Thus, the war may have created the conditions of possibility necessary for modern women to emerge, but it was postwar commercial beauty culture that provided the strategies and goods required to make women modern.

The notion that modern womanhood evolved in tandem with interwar consumer culture resonates among scholars who consider it a global development. Most recently, scholars working as part of the Modern Girl Around the World Research Group have demonstrated that modern women emerged simultaneously in the crowded corridors of Tokyo, in the bustling bazaars of Bombay, and on the glittering *grandes boulevards* of Paris.[5] Produced at the juncture of global economic structures and transnational cultural flows, the "Modern Girl" signified a "new form of femininity," one that "centered on purchased products for the body."[6] Connected not by nationality, race, language, or geography but rather by sex, age, appearance, "explicit eroticism," and the "use of specific commodities," the international Modern Girl became a privileged and charged "marker of modernity."[7] The Modern Girl, as both a contested cultural symbol and an anxiety-producing social phenomenon, constituted "either an object of celebration or of attempted control" in "all of the national contexts in which she appeared."[8] Indeed, across the globe, the Modern Girl engaged thorny debates regarding woman's morality, her controversial relationship to consumerism, and even her tenuous position within the nation.[9] These heated contests undeniably framed the contradictory lenses through which Modern Girls were seen at the same time that they signaled transnational concerns about feminine identity and visibility.

By examining the relationship between women and commercial beauty culture in interwar France, the chapters that follow contribute to and build upon the important findings uncovered by the Modern Girl Around the World Research Group. I, too, am interested in tracing the intersections between commodities and bodies, so central to the modern woman's self-production. Through the lens of beauty contests and cinema, chapter 5 explores the ways that commercial beauty culture facilitated the commodification of female bodies. Specifically, I investigate how, through the unapologetic display of cosmetically enhanced female bodies, these media legitimized the modern woman's desire for visibility at the same time that they created a new, consumable iconography of feminine beauty. Chapter 6 develops this line of inquiry further, examining the ways that the beauty industry encouraged women to identify with and to create identity through the cosmetic products that they purchased. By crafting packages that were as functional as they were decorative, making quality products accessible to discerning consumers, and providing technical, specialized advice, commercial beauty culture empowered women with the products and skills required to make their own beauty. Moreover, by emphasizing corporeal discipline, restraint, and self-control, messengers of this culture reiterated the aphorism that the pursuit of beauty remained an important form of women's work.

The chapters that follow also analyze the transnational cultural forms and commercial processes through which women were invented and presented as markers of modernity. Chapter 5 examines the emergence of modern women in two burgeoning popular entertainment venues, the beauty contest and the cinema. Amalgamations of French and international (primarily American) enterprises, pageants and films sanctioned the public display of female bodies and introduced standards of corporeal beauty that visually distinguished the "girl of today" from women of the past. As ordinary women strove to emulate sirens of stage and screen, commercial beauty culture, as chapter 6 demonstrates, stood at the ready to help them do so. Cosmetics firms, retailers, and beauty advisors not only provided tools and tips that enabled women to imitate the look of their icons, they also, through creative packaging and product design, innovative retailing, and advocacy of rational corporeal maintenance, coupled science with aesthetics to portray bodily care itself as modern.

Although much of what follows extends arguments advanced by the Modern Girl Around the World Research Group, I part ways with these scholars on two points. First, I differ with the group in regard to precise terminology. The group argues convincingly that the term *girl* "signifies the contested status of young women, no longer children, and their unstable and sometimes subversive relationships to social norms relating to heterosexuality, marriage, and motherhood" at the same time that it offers "a modern social and representational category" and a "style of self-expression largely delinked from biological age."[10] Both justifications for using the term are warranted; in fact, I use the concept of the "girl of today" in chapter 5 to analyze how modern womanhood developed through interwar cultural media; however, I interchange it with "woman" because contemporaries used both terms. Chapter 6, for example, begins with an excerpt from a beauty-manual author who addresses not the "girl of today," but "today's woman." By using both terms, my work endeavors to appropriately recognize the postwar decade's emphasis on youth while also acknowledging how historical actors viewed themselves.

Second, whereas the group found that in "all of the national contexts in which she appeared," the Modern Girl was "either an object of celebration or of attempted control," my study reveals how, in interwar France, these currents coexisted. Rather than posit a bifurcated response to modern womanhood, I show how the cinema starlet, the beauty contestant, and the imagined female consumer who enlivened beauty advertisements acted simultaneously as sites of celebration and contestation. Indeed, modern womanhood signaled contradiction, not conciliation, and that is why modern women fueled rather than resolved postwar debates regarding feminine visibility and identity. Moreover, exploring modern womanhood as a series of entangled contradictions exposes the extent to which debates about modern women upheld and destabilized gender norms; revealing in the process how, in the early decades of the twentieth century, cultural anxieties around modernity were consistently voiced in the language of the feminine.

5

Creating the "Girl of Today"

> Beauty, like everything else, comes quickly to an end, and I feel I must abandon my pretentious title. From America I have received many tempting offers, but I am afraid to go there, for they have so many beautiful women in America that I may appear to make claims which I cannot any longer make good.
>
> —Agnès Souret, La plus belle femme de France, 1920

In the spring of 1928, France and America were at war. Conflict erupted not on a desolate battlefield but on the picturesque beaches of Galveston, Texas. Combatants were not solemn men outfitted in uniforms and equipped with modern weapons but exuberant young women adorned in colorful bathing suits and armed only with the chief weapon in the coquette's arsenal—a dazzling smile. Indeed, that June, France and America did not encounter one another in the theater of war but instead were competing on the stage of the Third Annual "International Pageant of Pulchritude," also known as the Miss Universe Pageant. In the competition, which included forty-two contestants (thirty-two from the United States and ten of foreign origin), Miss France, Raymonde Allain, placed second behind Miss Chicago, Ella Van Hueson.[1] On the international pageant stage, contestants like Allain and Van Hueson were more than pretty girls vying for a title; they were also front-line soldiers in a transatlantic battle of cultures.

Unsurprisingly, in press coverage of the event, commentators distinguished contestants by evoking nationally specific definitions of feminine beauty. According to a *Washington Post* correspondent reporting from Paris, the pageant's significance resided in one deceptively simple question: "What constitutes real beauty?" Yet behind this question loomed a more complex, if subtler, problem: Was "real beauty" French, or was it American? On this issue, astonishingly, the cultural elite of Paris was divided. While Raymonde Allain was "heralded at home as a modern Venus" because she "possessed in marked degree all the qualities of real French charm and chic," several of her countrymen and -women believed that she did not stand a chance against "the American girl," who "represents the highest type of feminine beauty in all the world." Not everyone was convinced of the superiority of American beauty, however. The author Pierre Dominique complained that "American girls are strident, vulgar, without beauty of face or form or spirit. . . . They have no scruples, no morals, no more feminine charm than peasant girls who work all their lives in the field. . . . They are hipless, breastless beings only for sport and jazz music. In a word, they are barbarians." Although far less critical than Dominique, the Miss France pageant organizer Maurice de Waleffe nonetheless pointed out that the French beauty contestant "is not the flat-chested thin-legged Mercury . . . but a well-built sixteen-year-old girl of today."[2]

Insistence on national particularity, however, obscured important cultural similarities between these countries, especially as they pertained to attitudes about women. In both France and America, the beauty contestant engaged complex cultural debates regarding women's visibility, their relationship to the consumer market, and their place in the nation. Before 1914, these debates had emerged primarily through print media: in the pamphlets of natalists and suffragettes, the daily press, fiction, and self-help manuals. These media continued to thrive but were increasingly overshadowed by visual media after the war.[3] Glossy magazines supplemented articles and editorials devoted to feminine appearance and comportment with photographs, illustrations, and pictorial advertisements. In the days before the talkie, the cinema united scenery, props, fashions, cosmetics, actors and actresses in momentary collages, creating alternate realities wherein spectators could envision themselves as the stars on-screen. Beauty contests went even further; they not only put images of attractive women on view, they also invited ordinary women to exhibit their bodies. Through the impenitent public display of female bodies, the woman's magazine, the cinema, and the beauty contest provided visually rich cultural and commercial forums for staging diverse models of womanhood.

Agreeing upon one model of womanhood was no easy task, especially when the contest winner was charged with the responsibility of representing her community, her region, or her nation. The limited scholarly attention devoted to beauty contests has focused largely on how these events conveyed communal values and promoted particular forms of national identity.[4] Scholars have read the contestant's body allegorically as a gendered representation of the nation or, more generously, as the façade of an embodied subject who, through performance, imbued "'naturalness' into political constructs like 'nation' and 'citizen.'"[5] Scholars have also argued that by insisting that contestants be young and unmarried, contests promoted the idea that woman's greatest service to her nation rested in her capacity to reproduce its citizens.[6] As potential mothers, contestants assured social stability and solidified the boundaries of national belonging. Thus the beauty contestant was not only supposed to represent a respectable image of womanhood; the "girl of today" was also expected to embody a national ideal.

This chapter moves beyond discussions of woman's duty to the nation to examine how and why interwar beauty contests engendered transnational debates about feminine beauty, identity, and visibility. The first part demonstrates how the photographic contest helped legitimize the public display of female bodies at the same time that it taught bourgeois women how to "look." The second section explores how the 1928 Miss Universe competition produced models of womanhood that simultaneously assumed and resisted national identification. The final part analyzes the Studio Kino film *Prix de beauté* to reveal how French and American beauty standards converged and diverged in the cinematic portrayal of a fictitious Miss Europe.

In all these contexts—the photo contest, the beauty pageant, and the film—the beauty contestant's commodified body articulated cultural anxieties about feminine visibility. These venues offered ambitious young women what seemed to be desirable pathways to self-fulfillment, as well as opportunities for fame, wealth, and independence. But these possibilities came with costs. Contests curtailed woman's autonomy by encouraging entrants and spectators alike to equate female selfhood with the exhibited body. Contests also problematized woman's relationship to the nation. Contestants represented a locality at the same time that they were packaged as (inter)national brands. Articulating tensions between the real and the imagined, the parochial and the international, beauty contestants embodied the girl of today and put on display both the inherent contradictions and the striking commonalities in transnational conceptions of modern womanhood.

PHOTOGRAPHIC BEAUTIES

Glossy magazines provided an early, important, and reputable commercial vehicle for the public display of female bodies. These periodicals addressed a vast array of issues, ranging from politics, art, and society to the domestic arts, fashion, and self-care.[7] Included as well were features on celebrities and socialites, advice columns dedicated to etiquette and housewifery, and scores of advertisements for commercial products and services that promised to make the bourgeois woman's life complete. Through editorials, articles, advertisements, and the sponsoring of beauty contests, moreover, magazines like *Femina,* the *Ladies' Home Journal,* and *Vogue* shaped new definitions of beauty.[8]

French and American magazines followed different developmental trajectories, and American journals were more likely to be read by women of modest means; however, both identified physical appearance as a legitimate female concern. Filled with images of fashionable women and with articles that acquainted readers with the latest beauty trends, *Femina,* the *Ladies' Home Journal,* and *Vogue* portrayed beauty work as woman's duty. By the 1920s, *Femina* had morphed from a general society magazine marginally preoccupied with the development of young women into a full-fledged lifestyle guide. Brimming with photographs and lavish, hand-drawn illustrations depicting socialites in the latest fashions, *Femina,* as Francesca Berry explains, "emphasized fantasy over practicality, expression over information, and desire over need."[9] The *Ladies' Home Journal* débuted on February 16, 1883, as a single-page supplement to *Tribune and Farmer,* but by 1903, its circulation had grown to more than 1 million.[10] Under the editor Edward Bok, the *Journal* doubled in size from sixteen to thirty-two pages and envisioned an "ideal woman" who, "by her dress, manner, and, in every way," represented the "best in American womanhood."[11]

Perhaps the most notable magazine to cross over from America to France was *Vogue.* Launched in 1892 as a society journal that catered exclusively to New York City's elite, *Vogue* soon became a national and international sensation. After the magazine's purchase by Condé Nast in 1909, *Vogue* set out to seduce not only the New York socialite but also any "woman of fashion" by showcasing the latest sartorial trends from Paris.[12] *Vogue* made its French-language début in 1921. Like *Femina, Vogue* sold for 4 francs per issue in the 1920s, and its annual subscription rate increased from 65 francs in the 1920s to near 100 francs by the late 1930s.[13] An expensive indulgence, these magazines were certainly out of the reach of most working-class women. For example, the average provincial French female textile worker earned between 17 and 19 francs a day in 1922 and would have spent about 80 percent of her budget on food and clothing, leaving very little left over for magazines.[14] By the mid-1920s, moreover, French consumers paid 2.75 francs for bread, 4 francs for a shirt, and between 6.5 (Crème Simon) and 46.5 (Caron) francs for a box of rice powder.[15] Certainly, women could find fashion and beauty advice in less expensive publications. *La coiffure et les modes,* the supplement of *Coiffure de Paris* and predecessor to *Votre beauté,* cost 3.5 francs in the 1920s, and *Le petit echo de la mode,* a Catholic weekly that targeted the petty bourgeoisie, could be purchased for 25–60 centimes during the interwar period. Although women of modest means could not afford to regularly purchase elite magazines like *Vogue,* these magazines nevertheless established normative standards of fashion and beauty that women across the social spectrum aspired to achieve.[16]

Women's periodicals not only set standards of beauty and fashion; they also popularized photographic beauty contests. More commonplace in American periodicals than in French ones, these competitions appeared in mass-circulated dailies and were often sponsored by outside investors. For example, in 1888, the circus promoter Adam Forepaugh used national newspapers to search for the country's most beautiful woman. More than eleven thousand women submitted photos, all hoping to win the grand prize: ten thousand dollars and a role in Forepaugh's production of Thomas Moore's *Lellah Rookh.* Regional newspapers soon began conducting their own contests: in 1901, the *St. Louis Globe-Democrat* sought a representative for the Louisiana Purchase Exposition of 1902; in 1904, the *Denver Post* sought the most beautiful woman in Colorado; in 1905, the *San Francisco Examiner* sought the five most beautiful women in California; and, in that same year, local papers across the country competed to send delegates to the St. Louis Exposition.[17]

Women's magazines expanded the contest, making media-based beauty competitions more competitive for participants, more lucrative for winners, and more engaging for readers. In 1904, *Femina* reported on American beauty contests, and three years later, in September 1907, the journal participated in an international contest launched by the *Chicago Tribune. Femina*'s competition for the most beautiful woman explicitly excluded "les beautés professionnelles" and required that amateur contestants have a friend or family member submit a recent photo. Selected by an illustrious jury of journalists, photographers, and other beauty experts, winners would be featured in the journal and awarded prizes.[18] In 1911, the *Ladies' Home Journal* launched its own amateur contest. Its "Loveliest Girls in America Contest" sought the ten most beautiful girls in each of the five major regions of the country. The winner was to receive a trip to New York City and to have her portrait done by the graphic artist Charles Dana Gibson, creator of the famous Gibson Girl.[19]

Beauty contests grew appreciably throughout the first decades of the twentieth century, becoming even more widespread in the 1920s. In 1924, French *Vogue* sponsored a "best silhouette" contest that awarded ten finalists fifty thousand francs in prizes ranging from furs to tea sets to jewelry and cosmetics. Prospective contestants sent pencil-drawn silhouettes of their profile (from the neck up) along with their name and address. A jury of fourteen artists who regularly collaborated with the magazine was charged with narrowing the field to twenty contestants, whose profile silhouettes were then featured in the December edition. *Vogue* asked readers to send in postcards listing and ordering the ten silhouettes they most preferred. The winner and nine other finalists, chosen by *Vogue* readers, were revealed in the January issue.[20] In this way, the *Vogue* silhouette competition exemplified the dominant features of the twentieth-century photographic contest: it recruited participants from the public; it relied on the expertise of a professional jury (usually artists, coiffeurs, or fashion experts) but also incorporated the popular vote; and it lavished finalists with luxurious commercial prizes.

In addition to magazine-sponsored contests were those linked to commercial beauty firms. In 1929, *Comoedia* partnered with the Bichara firm for its "most beautiful eyes of Paris" campaign, and in 1931, *Femina* cosponsored a "concours de la Petite Reine" (little queen contest) in which the winner received a modeling contract.[21] In America, commercially sponsored contests resembled those advertised in French periodicals but addressed a broader audience. In 1925, for example, the Golden Brown Company invited customers to vote for the most beautiful African American woman via coupons inserted into cosmetic packages, while the Woodbury's firm advertised its contest, which welcomed "every type of American woman" regardless of age or class.[22] Alongside these contests were a growing number of competitions geared toward beauty workers. In 1927, *La coiffure de Paris* launched its "makeup and manicure contest" in which participants were allotted one hour and fifteen minutes to give a client a manicure and to make her over with cosmetics. The goal of the competition was to publicize the skills of professional aestheticians and salon workers in personal beautification rituals. The contest became so popular that it was expanded in 1931 to include international participants, and it incorporated a new event featuring the best Marcel perm.[23]

On both sides of the Atlantic, women's magazines provided national forums for the public display and critique of female bodies. Photographic beauty contests in particular illuminated the diverse ways in which the press manufactured and disseminated ideas of feminine beauty. Involving ordinary women at every stage, the 1920s magazine contest ostensibly taught women how to "look." As amateur contestants, women disciplined their bodies to conform to a modernist beauty aesthetic that celebrated thinness, good health, and youth. Moreover, by submitting images of their profiles, their hands, their hair, and their silhouettes for public inspection in exchange for beauty products and other prizes, magazine contests helped link feminine corporeal display to the commercial beauty market. As anonymous jurors and readers—sending in postcard rankings of participants and debating contestant qualities with friends—women learned to evaluate the female form using standardized criteria. By instituting specific eligibility requirements and offering their own commentary, magazines conditioned women to appreciate certain corporeal attributes and to disdain others. Finally, after assessing these competitors, women undoubtedly turned a critical eye upon themselves. They compared their own bodies to those of contestants, they scrutinized their features for imperfections, and they invested in health and beauty aids in their own pursuit of the "look." Through the public display of female bodies, then, the photographic beauty contest legitimized the female gaze, transformed the most obscure hometown girls into national beauty icons, and indulged the girl of today's desire to see and to be seen. Contests, however, also linked beauty and commerce, elevated appearance over substance, and promoted an idealized model of womanhood that was presented as both performative and purchasable.

CREATING AND CROWNING THE "MISS"

Like the photographic competition, the beauty pageant provided an occasion for the public display of female bodies. At a moment when respectable women were becoming more visible on the public stage—as consumers, employees, social reformers, and students—the pageant stage offered a popular forum for debating modern womanhood.[24] Through the commodified female body, pageants like Miss France, Miss America, and Miss Universe incited cultural debates while acting as sites of cultural transfer and commercial exchange.

On the one hand, national and international pageants mobilized the female body as an emblem of national identity; on the other, they created a universal "Miss" whose value resided in her ability to elide national differences.

In the first decades of the twentieth century, beauty pageants evolved from local, small-scale amusements into national, large-scale commercial entertainments. Contests originated not as stand-alone events, but as attractions linked to popular civic festivals. By the 1920s, however, pageants attracted shrewd entrepreneurs who transformed them from primarily civic events into lucrative commercial spectacles. Investors sanitized the pageant image, making them respectable by implementing rigid eligibility criteria designed to attract only modest young women and by moving the contest beyond the circus and the carnival to establish it as an event in its own right.[25]

France had long celebrated feminine beauty by anointing "queens" at Lenten Festivals and Bastille Day events.[26] At the turn of the century, one of the most popular of these festivals was the Fête de la couronnement de la muse du peuple (Festival of the Crowning of the People's Muse). The fête became a major feature of many provincial and national civic celebrations from its first staging in 1897. The original People's Muse was a young laundress chosen by her peers to participate in the third act of the composer Gustave Charpentier's musical ceremony at the finale of Montmartre's Vache enragée (Carnival of the Raging Cow). The event was such a hit that it quickly spread throughout provincial fairs: it was performed in Lille in 1898; in Bordeaux in 1899; and in Le Mans and Rouen in 1900. The festival grew to include elaborate processionals featuring ostentatiously decorated floats, ceremonies with delegations of civic dignitaries, and decadent champagne toasts at city halls.[27]

As the contest's popularity increased, so did municipal and public interest in the muse. The contest became standardized: selection committees were no longer ad hoc assemblages of townspeople, but appointed officials with local notoriety. Strict rules for contestants were put into place—prospective participants had to be between the ages of sixteen and twenty-one, physically attractive, unmarried, and certifiably virtuous. Given her precarious class status—many contestants, like the laundress, came from humble origins—a woman's virtue became a particularly salient feature of the contest criteria. As the historian David Pomfret explains, local police were routinely called out to interview neighbors and companions to verify that contestants had not engaged in promiscuous activities.[28] Intended to represent the values of the republic, the muse garnered public recognition and achieved a certain amount of social capital within her community. However, as the winner of a contest, she also received prizes—clothing, small pieces of jewelry, and beauty products—provided by local merchants. Newspapers further facilitated the muse's commodification, publishing her picture for public consumption and printing her image for purchase. The intention of the fête may have been to promote the image of a youthful, virtuous France, but the contest also demonstrated how, through support for and interest in the beauty contest, contemporaries spectacularized and commodified feminine beauty in the decade before the Great War.

American pageants, too, were initially part of larger fairs. As early as the seventeenth century, women competed in New Orleans to be crowned Mardi Gras Queen, and American women had long vied for top honors at town festivals and May Day celebrations. By the twentieth century, beauty contests were regular features of carnivals and regional fairs. New York City's Easter Festival in 1900 included several beauty contests, and the St. Louis Exposition in 1905 featured young women from across the country representing their hometowns for the first time on a national stage. The origins of the first independent American beauty pageant are contested—some attribute the invention to P. T. Barnum in 1854; others cite the short-lived Miss United States contest that began in 1880. Scholars and pageant enthusiasts, however, agree that the modern pageant came into its own in September 1921, on the Atlantic City Boardwalk.[29]

Concerned about the exodus of tourists (and tourist dollars) after Labor Day, the hotel owner H. Conrad Eckholm convinced the Atlantic City Business Men's League that hosting a pageant would be a profitable way to extend the summer holiday season.[30] Included originally as part of the city's five-day Fall Frolic, the "Inter-City Beauty Pageant," or "Autumn Beauty Contest," as it was called, drew a modest number of contestants but attracted a crowd of more than one hundred thousand spectators. Despite rather strict rules—contestants could not be celebrities or have bobbed hair or wear visible makeup (this would make them appear too worldly)—the highlight of the event was the somewhat scandalous bathing-suit competition. Selected by audience applause, the winner, sixteen-year-old Margaret Gorman, received both a monetary prize and the now-famous mermaid trophy. On the heels of this success, the competition resumed the next year under its new name, the Miss America Pageant. Throughout the 1920s, the Miss America Pageant expanded, attracting a growing number of contestants and spectators and adding a panel of expert judges who evaluated contestants using increasingly standardized rules. Contestant height, weight, and measurements had to be within a certain range; age, race, and marital status became a formal part of the contest's eligibility criteria; and winners were prohibited from entering future contests.

Meanwhile, the Parisian journalist Maurice de Waleffe launched a concours de la plus belle femme de France in 1920.[31] De Waleffe's pageant shared many similarities with American contests, but instead of launching it as part of a civic celebration, the promoter capitalized on the thriving commercial entertainment market and held the contest in the movie houses of Paris. Forty-nine pageant contestants were divided up into seven groups of seven and trotted out to movie houses across the city, where theatergoers selected the most beautiful woman. The winner of the first contest, Agnès Souret, the seventeen-year-old daughter of a country lawyer, earned an astounding 114,994 votes.[32] Consequently, Souret's status as "the most beautiful woman in France" won her numerous show-business offers, including one from the Barnum Company to tour the United States.[33] After her victory, Souret posed for motion-picture stills and even appeared in the feature film *The Lily of Mont St. Michel*. Her life transformed virtually overnight as there was nowhere that she could go without being photographed or approached by adoring fans. So widespread was her fame, in fact, that "when she went shopping she was forced to wear a thick veil and goggles to escape being mobbed, and at the theatre door she needed a police escort through the crowd of would-be swains."[34] Exhausted and overcome by all of the attention paid her, Souret retired from public life within two years of winning her title. She was nineteen years old.

De Waleffe's pageant differed from its American counterparts, however, in its ideological scope. Concerned about the war's effects on French society, the successful journalist intended that his pageant produce "ethnically French" models of womanhood that would restore gender norms and racial order. Although open to women born to foreign parents and eventually (in the 1930s Miss France d'Outre-Mer contests) to colonial participants, de Waleffe's vision of ethnically French womanhood was decidedly white and provincial. De Waleffe believed that the physically robust and healthfully fertile provincial woman offered a much-needed antidote to urban degeneration, overcivilization, and national decline. Charged with rejuvenating the French race, the beauty queen signaled a return to the parochial and patriarchal. Yet as herself the product of a media-driven consumerist enterprise, she could not be divorced from the modern, industrial world that created her. Indeed, despite efforts to celebrate natural feminine beauty—a curvaceous figure, unblemished, sun-kissed skin—contestants showed up to the 1920s pageant sporting the latest figure-trimming fashions and covered in makeup. Winner Agnès Souret embodied this paradox between tradition and modernity when she was photographed in modest provincial garb for certain publications and in risqué cabaret attire for others. Blending the provincial and the urban, the preindustrial and the consumerist, Souret ultimately posed more questions about racial order and gender norms than she answered.[35]

At the same time that de Waleffe launched his plus belle femme de France competition, an American entrepreneur began organizing a contest that would become the world's first international beauty pageant. In 1920, C. E. Barfield planned an event that would bring tourists back to the Texas seaside. That year, he introduced "Splash Day," which featured a "Bathing Girl Revue" as its main attraction. The event took place at the beginning of summer, thus not extending but kicking off the tourist season. Its popularity swelled throughout the 1920s, and the competition soon became known outside of Texas. By 1926, Barfield's little contest had evolved into the world's first global beauty contest, the International Pageant of Pulchritude.[36] The original competition included thirty-nine entrants, thirty-seven from the United States and two of foreign origin (Mexico and Canada). In 1927, contestants for the Miss Universe Pageant were still primarily American (representing twenty-nine states), but eight foreign countries, including France, were invited to send delegates.[37]

In response to this invitation, de Waleffe initiated a Miss France contest.[38] This contest combined elements from earlier French competitions and from the Miss America Pageant. For example, participants were required to be French (i.e., born to French mothers), to be between the age of sixteen and twenty-five, to have never married, and to have never been employed by any business in the entertainment industry, specifically, the theater, the music hall, or the cinema. As in the Miss America Pageant, Miss France contestants paraded the runway clothed only in bathing suits, showing off their youthful figures to an audience that now included a special panel of "expert" judges. Hundreds of women applied to compete, but it was only the contest winner, Roberte Cusey, a young woman from the Jura, who was invited to Galveston. Cusey placed eighth (seventh runner-up) in the Miss Universe contest, but retained her title as the first official Miss France.

The stakes were higher the following year, when a stunning sixteen-year-old Breton named Raymonde Allain captured the Miss France title. Born into a respectable family, Allain was a relatively unknown teenager when she entered the contest. The pageant stage, however, elevated her to the public stage, transforming the amateur beauty into an overnight *femme célèbre*. From the moment of victory, reporters assiduously documented every part of Allain's pageant journey, publishing daily accounts of her activities, turning every aspect of her life into a media spectacle.[39] Journals highlighted different aspects of the pageant. *Le journal* focused on facts and details of the trip. *Le figaro* speculated on the link between female beauty and woman's domestic role. *Illustration* celebrated the competitive aspects of the pageant—comparing the event to a boxing match! However, each story was packaged so as to communicate the "pageant experience," and each image of Allain was intended to publicize a certain vision of French feminine beauty. For, as the reigning Miss France, Allain was not only a commodified beauty queen; she was also becoming an international symbol of French womanhood and an ambassador of the French nation.

When Allain arrived in Galveston with seven other foreign competitors at Pier 20 on June 1, they were "accorded a welcoming ovation by several thousand persons."[40] Three days later, an estimated 150,000 spectators arrived by boat, car, and eighteen specially designated trains to observe the opening parade.[41] The newspaperman Stanley Babb reported that it was in "high carnival humor" that spectators clamored to glimpse the "charming maidens gathered together from the four corners of the world."[42] Festivities continued the next day, culminating in the penultimate portion of the event, the crowning of Miss United States from the field of American competitors. The winner was Miss Chicago, a twenty-two-year-old named Ella Van Hueson. Still celebrating her victory, Van Hueson joined her forty-one rivals onstage for the Miss Universe competition on the evening of June 6. A jury of seven men, including the comic-book artist Harry Tuthill from Missouri, the sculptor Albert Reiker from New Orleans, and the portrait and theater artist W. V. Guinness from Philadelphia, watched from within the crowd as contestants paraded on the stage first in the latest gowns from Paris and then in bathing suits recently purchased in a Galveston department store.[43] Although the "modest and retiring type," Miss France came alive onstage, unfolding "like a rose" so that her "sweet smile captured every heart." Yet even her sweet smile could not overcome the "charmingly tactful and gracious" beauty of Ella Van Hueson (see fig. 5.1).[44]

Commentators used the 1928 Miss Universe competition to attribute national characteristics to the displayed female bodies. Through the figures of

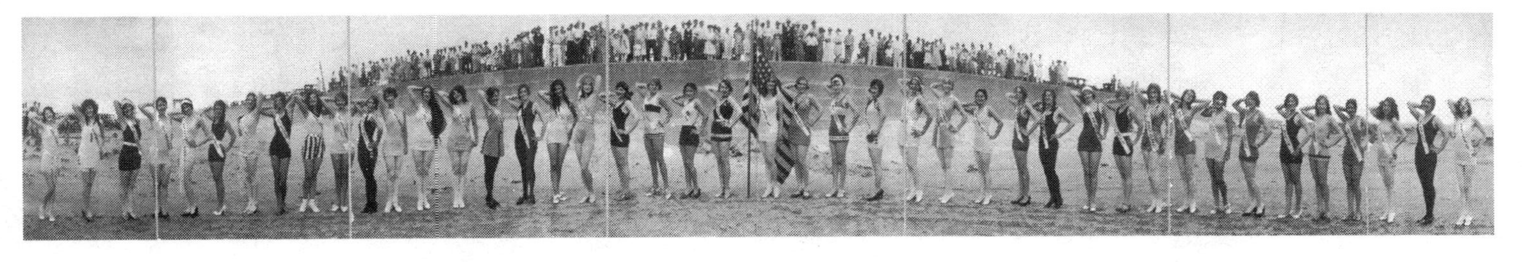

Fig. 5.1. Third International Pageant of Pulchritude and Ninth Annual Bathing Girl Revue. Galveston, Texas. Courtesy of Library of Congress.

Raymonde Allain and Ella Van Hueson, French "chic and charm" went head-to-head with the "academic perfection of the American type."[45] Maurice de Waleffe explained to the *Washington Post* that the "girl who represents France was more than plastic beauty." She "has charm of personality, a certain French vivaciousness of expression and a body which should inspire great modern artists." Allain, according to de Waleffe, epitomized all of this and more. Not only was she a "living, breathing young person of culture," but she was also "a virginal nymph [who] sprung from the best of French stock." Conversely, the "golden-haired" Van Hueson embodied the "American standard of girlhood physically." Maître Paul Chebas, former president of the Académie des beaux arts and member of the Miss France jury that elected Allain, acknowledged that "American girls are goddesses of health and beauty. As such they are hard to beat. I have been watching them for the last twenty years in my studio, at the theaters, on the boulevards, and I have come to the conclusion that they are truly Olympian in their physical perfection." Another jury member, the esteemed Parisian dressmaker Jenny, explained: "There are very few defects in the shapes of American girls. . . . If an American woman is beautiful and also possesses that subtle thing called personality, there is no mortal being that can compete with her."[46] Possessing both beauty and personality, Ella Van Hueson, not Raymonde Allain, won the grand prize: two thousand dollars, a silver plaque, and the coveted Miss Universe title.

Van Hueson and Allain entered into a complicated cultural contest when they agreed to compete in the Miss Universe pageant. Within their own national contexts, both women exemplified a certain kind of idealized beauty, and through this embodiment they offered safe alternatives to the menacing flapper and to the transgressive *garçonne*. Yet on the international pageant stage, they competed not against their antitheses but against women who epitomized this same kind of beauty. The sculptress who modeled Allain, Anna Bess, drew comparisons to the contestants, acknowledging that Allain's "sweet form reflects the wonderful carving of a healthy occupation. She is so much like an American in that respect."[47] At five feet six-and-a-half inches and 120 pounds, Van Hueson exemplified the image of the "fit" American, and although she was six years older than Allain, commentators noted her youthfulness.[48] Whereas age and physicality reinforced one another on the body of Van Hueson, they appeared somehow at odds on the countenance of Allain. In her face, Bess noted "all her grace, hidden and visible, how powerfully organized for the perplexities of modern times."[49] The distinction here was both subtle and illuminating. American beauty, as represented by Van Hueson, was admirable in its physical fitness as well as in its youthful vigor. It was, as so many French commentators referred to it, a "plastic perfection." Allain's beauty, also radiant in its corporeal exuberance, was subdued, contemplative, connected to her charm and to her comportment as a "person of culture." What emerged from a comparison of Van Hueson and Allain was the message that although beauty contestants shared a variety of similar characteristics, ideal beauty itself meant something very different in America and France in the 1920s.

From 1928 on, France hosted a Miss France Pageant and sent a delegate to the Miss Universe competition.[50] Throughout the twentieth century, Miss France and her counterparts, Miss United States and Miss America, have served as national icons of femininity and beauty. At the same time as these women have personified the aesthetic values of their *patrie,* however, they also embodied an international beauty ideal that was young, slender, white, and seemingly classless. Miss America's "plastic perfection" and Miss France's "chic and charm" indicated national preferences, but at any moment one model of beauty could prevail over the other; Miss Universe could be "plastic" one year and "chic" the next. As a participant in (and sometimes winner of) the Miss Universe Pageant, these women embodied both competing and universal ideals of feminine beauty.

It is precisely in this capacity to both reinforce and resist national identifications, to be both national symbol and international icon, that the beauty queen transformed from an ordinary woman into a transnational beauty commodity. In the early stages of the competition, the media and pageant sponsors highlighted the personal histories and personalities of pageant contestants; yet, once the "Miss" was crowned, the individual's private identity was obscured behind the title, and Miss France/America the woman was eclipsed by Miss France/America the brand. Thus, through the pageant process the female body was simultaneously spectacularized and objectified, packaged as a national commodity and venerated as an international, mass ornament.

PRIX DE BEAUTÉ

As the interwar pageant queen endeavored to solidify her status as a transnational beauty icon, she increasingly shared that spotlight with a new formidable opponent—the cinema starlet. Indeed, homegrown celebrities were often eclipsed by ultraglamorous Hollywood ingénues who entered France first through silent films and then through talkies. The Hollywood machine intentionally promoted actresses to embody specific types of beauty—the girl next door, the femme fatale, the modern girl. Confronted with images of women with whom they identified or whose image they aspired to replicate, female theatergoers were eager to learn about their idols, especially how these women achieved their "look." The camera close-up called attention to the celebrity's skin, to her expression, and to her makeup. Conveniently, product tie-ins within films and as advertisements played before screenings and during double-feature intermissions introduced spectators to products that could help them achieve the look that they admired on-screen.[51]

Women's periodicals picked up where cinema advertisements left off. *Femina, Vogue, Votre beauté,* and other society magazines had long associated celebrity with beauty (recall the Grand Coquettes). From the late nineteenth century forward, they employed performers to contribute beauty columns, cited them as models worthy of emulation, and published countless stories about their private lives. In 1932, Juliette Goublet (the same reporter who had covered the opening of Colette's beauty institute) revisited music-hall performer–turned–cinema siren Cécile Sorel in an article for *Beauté-coiffure-mode.* After discussing aesthetic standards and acknowledging her appreciation of the corporeal beauty of classical Greece, Sorel offered this advice: "A pretty woman is sober, sleeps a lot, does not take too much alcohol or red meat, and practices sport, especially walking."[52]

Magazines also upheld celebrities, like the notorious Belle Époque stage performer– turned-courtesan Liane de Pougy as models of feminine beauty and charm. In her own diary entry from August 24, 1919 (when the actress was past her prime), Pougy described her physical portrait: "Tall and looking even more so," she wrote, "1.66 meters, 56 kilos in my clothes. I run to length—long neck, face a full oval but elongated, pretty well perfect, long arms, long legs." She then explained that her complexion was "pale and matte, skin very fine. I use the merest touch of rouge, it suits me. Rather small mouth, well shaped, superb teeth. My nose? They say it's the marvel of marvels." After describing her "pretty little ears," she confided that she had "almost no eyebrows—hence a little pencil whenever I want it. Eyes a green hazel, prettily shaped, not very large—but my look is large. Hair thick and very fine, incredibly fine, a pretty shiny chestnut brown. Hardly any grey hairs. One or two to prove that I don't dye."[53] Renowned as an extraordinary beauty, Pougy's intimate self-portrait revealed the corporeal aesthetic standards of her day: long, thin body; pale, refined skin exhibiting the slightest hint of color; well-shaped features; and luxurious hair.

Magazines attempted to provide similarly intimate knowledge about celebrities by publishing stories about their private lives. Often these stories were part of the celebrity's own public relations campaign or turned out to be little more than gossip collected from self-proclaimed insiders. The opera singer and international beauty icon Caroline "la belle" Otero addressed the press's penchant for spreading gossip in her own 1927 memoir: "There is nothing on earth so likely to set people talking about you as to ignore everything they say and tell them nothing on your own account. To this day, when I have left the stage there are still rumours floating about. Quite lately, I had a telephone inquiry from a lady who wished to know where I had had the facial operation done that had restored to me my looks as they were at twenty. I have never undergone this operation and I never shall undergo it."[54]

Given their obsession with European celebrities, it is not surprising that the French media and French audiences adored Hollywood actresses. In 1932, *Votre beauté* made Carole Lombard its cover girl one month and gave Judith Wood its cover for another. Three years later, the magazine ran a story entitled "To Be Beautiful Like a Star," in which the contributor detailed the beauty routines of Joan Crawford, Katherine Hepburn, Jean Harlow, and Lombard. And, in a 1936 article entitled "Hollywood Stars Pass as Beauty Models," *Votre beauté* included pictures and discussed the beauty secrets of Marlene Dietrich, Crawford, Jeanette MacDonald, and Greta Garbo.[55] *Votre beauté* was not alone in its admiration of Hollywood stars. *Femina* sought the "counsel of Mlle. Fanny Ward" in 1929,[56] sending a staff writer to accompany the actress to her Paris spa treatment. The author dutifully recorded the process and provided hand-drawn pictures of the actress's hot oil bath, facial, and eyebrow plucking. Similarly, *Pour vous!* dedicated an article to "makeup in ten minutes" that featured not a Parisian socialite or French celebrity, but a photo of Ginger Rogers applying powder at her studio vanity.[57]

Audiences not only wanted to know the beauty secrets of Hollywood stars; they also wanted to use the same products. In 1926, Fanny Ward opened "The Fountain of Youth," a beauty shop in Paris; in 1930, Gloria Swanson and Constance Bennet introduced their own cosmetics line; the French brand "Madame Ouvry" launched its "masque de Hollywood," and French consumers demanded Max Factor cosmetics.[58] In 1938, *Votre beauté* showed the makeup artist as he transformed an ordinary woman into a star with nothing but skill and face paints.[59] Not surprisingly, it was during the 1930s that Max Factor began selling his "movie star makeup" to ordinary women. The September 1936 issue of *Vogue,* for example, ran an ad for Factor products entitled "Secrets de stars," which featured Bette Davis applying powder from a Max Factor compact and Claudette Colbert covering her lips with dark-red Max Factor lipstick.[60] Max Factor makeup and Hollywood features that shamelessly promoted American beauty products with product tie-ins, and on-screen advertisements bombarded moviegoers with new images of feminine beauty and with new methods for achieving it.[61] If one wanted to emulate the angelic beauty of Jean Harlow, for example, one had only to purchase the right brand of platinum-blond hair dye.

Desiring to look like the Hollywood actresses on-screen, female spectators purchased products that enabled them to make spectacles of themselves. In this way, spectators not only consumed the actresses as commodities and conflated image with identity, they also saw themselves as engaged in the performance of femininity. If the cinema was, as Richard Kuisel claims, a "force that standardized people," and the "quintessential expression of American culture," then Hollywood actresses threatened to homogenize French beauty and to turn French spectators into American-style consumers in one fell swoop.[62] Although French women undeniably desired to look like Hollywood starlets and Hollywood certainly provided the French public with a wide variety of American beauties to emulate, the American movie machine did not simply co-opt or colonize France's commercial beauty culture. In fact, the relationship between the two underwent continuous negotiation throughout the interwar period.

The Italian film pioneer Augusto Genina's feature-length *Prix de beauté* exemplified how American and French commercial and cultural interests both competed and intermingled. The beauty contestant and the cinema starlet converged in the film's protagonist, the petite-bourgeois secretary Lucienne Garnier, played by the American actress Louise Brooks. Lucienne resembles her coworkers: her dresses are fashionably cut and tailored to her figure; her hair is cropped in the popular bob style; and she wears cosmetics.[63] But Lucienne is not content to merely fit in; she craves attention and social mobility. She obsessively compares herself to women in fashion magazines and imagines appearing in the society pages of the *Globe,* the newspaper that employs her.

When the newspaper sponsors a beauty contest, Lucienne seizes the opportunity and, against her fiancé's wishes, submits her photo. Although Lucienne has been working under the supervision of the *Globe*'s editors for years, she only becomes visible to them through her contest photograph. Her visibility, of course, is contingent upon her physical beauty. It is Lucienne's stunning facial features, not her skillful typing, that attracts the notice of the all-male editorial jury. After reviewing hundreds of photos, the jury unanimously selects Lucienne to represent France in the Miss Europe Pageant.

Genina's camera captures the excitement of the pageant, panning to the numerous spectators in attendance before moving backstage to expose the fragmented female bodies (legs with stockings, bare shoulders, partially made-up faces) of the pageant contestants. Portraying contestants as an assortment of broken bodies, the camera simultaneously individualized and obscured the identities of the beauty contestants themselves.[64] By reducing contestants to their physical characteristics, the film suggests that beautiful women are composed of legs, arms, faces, and torsos that work together to create one harmonious template. Thus it is the collection of desirable physical attributes, as well as a woman's unique "personality," that together constitute the spectacle. Next, the camera pans to the stage where contestants parade the runway clad only in bathing suits and high-heeled shoes, subject to whistles, stares, and audience applause.[65] Participants are admired for both their difference from and similarity to one another: they may be blond, brunette, short, or tall, but all are well-built, young, and beautiful.

On the pageant stage, Lucienne easily charms spectators with her seductive walk and appealing physique. By audience applause she wins the Miss Europe Pageant. Like real-life pageant winners, Lucienne is lavished with expensive prizes (a new wardrobe, furs, jewelry); she becomes an overnight celebrity; and, posing for photographs, she participates in the commodification of her own image. Through the Miss Europe contest, Lucienne finally achieves the recognition that she so desperately desired while isolated in the secretarial pool. Yet Lucienne's enjoyment is short-lived. Distraught when he learns that she has competed in the pageant, her suitor André impetuously proposes marriage. Lucienne is torn between pursuing a domestic life with André and capitalizing on her fame to launch a career in cinema.

Choosing between a life of respectable domesticity and indulgent celebrity was a common dilemma for beauty contestants, and it is this choice that structures the dramatic tension in *Prix de beauté*. Although pageant organizers instituted strict rules prohibiting professional beauties and morally suspect women from entering, they could not control the decisions that contestants made once the competition ended. In fact, beauty contestants were often inundated with movie deals, theater offers, and modeling contracts. For example, all eight foreign competitors in the 1928 Miss Universe Pageant were propositioned before they left Galveston. Winner Ella Van Hueson was known to have entertained a "large number of theatrical offers."[66] Yet the opportunity to pursue a career in the entertainment industry seemed at odds with the Miss Universe Pageant's unspoken agenda of promoting a socially acceptable, morally adroit model of womanhood. How could the beauty queen reproduce the nation if, rather than returning to the foyer, she succumbed to her own desires? By pursuing her own pleasures, moreover, was she not coming dangerously close to resembling the hedonistic flapper and the childless *garçonne*?

Lucienne initially chooses respectability over fame and fortune. Foregoing her publicity tour, she marries André and sets up house in Paris. Returning to the monotony of her precelebrity existence, Lucienne is now trapped in a claustrophobic newlywed apartment rather than in the secretarial pool. With no outside employment, Lucienne resembles the caged canary hanging in the window of her flat, her days punctuated only by the comings and goings of her neighbors and her husband, who treats her like his own caged bird. Indeed, the scenes depicting Lucienne's married life are bleak: she prepares lunch and keeps house with sadness etched into her face; she sings sad songs to her avian companion; she counts the minutes of her passing youth with the incessant chirping of a wall-mounted cuckoo clock; and she dines morosely with André, who cunningly conceals letters that arrive addressed to "Miss Europe."

Despite her acquiescence, however, Lucienne remains, as evidenced by her cropped hair, trim silhouette, and obvious dissatisfaction with domestic monotony, a modern woman. Indeed, she is ultimately rescued from her domestic fate when one afternoon a stranger knocks on her door. The dapper middle-aged visitor informs Lucienne that he is a representative of the Sound Film International group. The group, he tells her, saw her film tests from San Sebastian and wants to contract her to star in feature films. At first, Lucienne rips up the contract. But as the day progresses, she changes her mind, opting to leave André and the tedium of domesticity to pursue the public life of a movie star.

The last scene of the film marks Lucienne's cinematic début. Watching a private test screening of her new feature, Lucienne appears in an evening gown alongside the producer who has vowed to make her famous. Enraptured by her own performance on the screen, she welcomes the producer's hand on her own and never sees the jealous, heartbroken André break into the theater. Disheveled and visibly distraught, André stares at Lucienne first in the audience and then on-screen. Overcome with emotion, he pulls a pistol from his front coat pocket, aims, and kills the beauty queen with one shot. The film ends with Lucienne's movie playing on over the cinema screen, casting shadows over the dead woman's lifeless face. The theater reverberates with Lucienne's sweet voice singing about her tortured life as a glamorous Venus.[67]

Precariously positioned between two competing visions of modernity, one domestic, predictable, and banal, the other public, capricious, and exhilarating, Lucienne's death is all but inevitable. Yet Lucienne does not find herself in this position because she is a typist, a housewife, or even a modern woman, but because she has won a beauty contest. Winning Miss Europe transforms Lucienne from an ordinary young woman into an awe-inspiring Venus. And it is this victory that places her in a most tenuous position. After she wins the competition, her personal freedom is curtailed by the contradictory expectations placed upon the "Miss." On the one hand, the respectable Miss was expected to return to the foyer to biologically and metaphorically reproduce. The docile body of the youthful pageant princess was in a state of becoming, only starting to mature; it could therefore be harnessed, disciplined for motherhood in a way that could effectively put the single modern woman in her place.[68] On the other hand, the glamorous Miss was supposed to represent an idyllic standard of feminine beauty, and it was her duty to share this perfection with the public through performance and display. The Miss, in this assessment, was nothing less than a collectively owned commodity, a woman who belonged not to herself but to a public that admired her.[69]

For Lucienne, there was no compromise between these positions. Forced to choose between domesticity and celebrity, she inevitably fulfilled one set of expectations while eschewing another. In this scenario, it is not only, as some feminist film critics have argued, modernity or a masculine fear of modernity that kills the beauty queen, but an irresolvable tension between competing ideals of modern womanhood that ensures her demise.[70] As Miss Europe—as a woman positioned between convention and fame—Lucienne is simultaneously granted and denied the liberation she desires. Because she belongs to everyone else, she loses herself. In her death, then, the beauty prize has been purchased at the ultimate price: Miss Europe the woman has been sacrificed to Miss Europe the ideal.

Lucienne's peculiar liminality is expertly foreshadowed from the beginning of the movie by the filmmaker's selection of the American actress Louise Brooks to play a French woman who becomes Miss Europe. It is notable that in a film featuring an all-French cast, an American actress plays the main character. Why would Genina intentionally cast an American to portray a French beauty queen? Louise Brooks was a known entity: she was already recognized internationally as a talented performer, famous for her European roles; and, as her costar René Clair explained, she also possessed "all of the qualities of physical beauty required for the role."[71] Yet casting an American had important cultural implications. As both the fictitious Miss Europe and as the star of a French film, Brooks embodied an ideal feminine beauty that was both particular and generic. Certainly, Brooks represented only one version of female beauty—young, thin, modern, American. However, by portraying a French Miss Europe, she also promoted a standardized type of feminine beauty that blended French and American ideals. In this way, Brooks embodied a feminine beauty aesthetic that transcended national borders, and *Prix de beauté* presented the beauty contest as a dynamic site of cross-cultural commercial exchange. The selection of Brooks as the leading lady thus verified how issues of national identity could be mutually framed and contested through venues that united female performance and commercial spectacle.

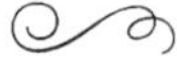

Far more than frivolous amusements or trivial popular entertainments, beauty contests illuminated the salient contradictions that underwrote productions of modern womanhood. Inasmuch as she epitomized the wholesome "girl of today," the beauty queen proposed a socially suitable corrective to the androgynous and promiscuous women visible in the jazz clubs of Paris and on the streets of New York City. Despite the contest's emphasis on wholesomeness, however, the contestant was still expected to fulfill her destiny as a desirable Venus. Ironically, in her postcontest pursuit of celebrity, the contestant grew to resemble the independent women who had served as her foil. Transforming the pure, innocent girl of today into the seductive, worldly modern woman, the beauty contest acted as a privileged register for the decade's fluctuating definitions of womanhood.

Beauty contests also exposed how commercial and cultural forces together produced models of womanhood. Calling attention to women's bodies and promoting the idea that identity could be purchased along with the latest fashions, women's magazines offered commercialized but socially acceptable forums for feminine display. Soliciting reader photos and opinions for their photographic contests, periodicals helped legitimize public scrutiny of the female form and proposed a model of respectable womanhood that elevated appearance over substance. On the pageant stage, young women eagerly subjected their bodies to both the gaze of the mixed-sex crowd as well as to its comment. Yet even this activity could be considered reputable as long as the contestant signified something greater than herself—her city, her region, or her nation. In its depiction of the fictitious Miss Europe, *Prix de beauté* exposed the hidden tension between representation and embodiment with which beauty contestants struggled. The film further complicated this tension by exploiting a series of misidentifications: playing Miss Europe, Brooks the actress used her own commodified (and American) body to represent a cross-cultural (American and French) beauty ideal. As Miss Europe, Brooks is French *and* American at the same time that she is *neither* French *nor* American. Brooks, like Miss Europe, is paradoxically local and global; real and imagined; consumer and consumed.

By engaging the question of whether "real beauty," as the *Washington Post* reporter called it, was French or American, beauty contests divulged how ideals of feminine beauty simultaneously reinforced and subverted national particularities. On the surface, feminine beauty in the 1920s appeared decidedly American: an American won the Miss Universe Pageant not only in 1928 but also in 1926, 1927, and 1930; and, an American actress rather than a French one was cast to portray the French Miss Europe. But rather than indicate America's growing hegemony over international beauty standards, this chapter has read examples like these as transatlantic cultural transfers between two countries for whom the female body symbolized and subverted national identifications. The French embraced Brooks less for her American look than for her "international style."[72] And, although Van Hueson bested Allain in the Miss Universe Pageant, commentators never suggested that Allain was inferior to Van Hueson, only that the women offered two different images of womanhood. In so doing, Allain and Van Hueson signified national beauty standards at the same time that they represented transnational beauty ideals.

The photographic beauty, the Miss, and the cinematic portrayal of Miss Europe illustrate the many ways that femininity was produced through the visual in the interwar period. By publicly displaying the female body, beauty contests celebrated diverse facets of modern womanhood: youth, innocence, sexuality, worldliness. As mass commodities, beauty contestants submitted their bodies to represent the nation or to embody a commercial brand like Miss Universe. In this way, contests generated female images that were as transitory and fleeting as the modern woman herself. The beauty contestant ultimately played multiple roles concurrently: disembodied spectacle *and* embodied symbol; national icon *and* transnational commodity. Through these multifaceted performances, the beauty contestant epitomized the contradictions and the cultural tensions that woman's visibility manifested in creating the girl of today.

6

Making Beauty Modern

> Today's woman, active, sporty, and who by the demands of modern life is called upon to be clothed in a manner that is comfortable, practical, even somewhat masculine, must acquire through makeup a healthy and natural beauty. . . . Sentimentality is no longer in season. It is important to live honestly, hygienically, without any constraint.
>
> —Madame Phyllis Earle, *Vogue,* December 1927

Identifying "today's woman" as "active," "sporty," and "practical," the *Vogue* contributor Phyllis Earle distinguished her from the "sentimental" woman of the past. In the 1920s, she declared, "to follow fashion takes more than 'arranging' one's face." Indeed, to live "honestly, hygienically," and "without any constraint," woman had to abandon the frivolity associated with the "outdated toilette of yesteryear" and cast aside once and for all "the frilly lace that gave woman the fragile appearance of a doll."[1] As Earle portrayed her, today's woman not only discarded outmoded practices and fashions, she also adopted a decidedly more pragmatic attitude about, and approach toward, bodily care. No longer satisfied with embodying the pleasing, passive, decorative object, the "active" woman mobilized the tools of France's commercial beauty culture to pursue a "healthy and natural beauty."

The cosmetics manufacturers, retailers, and self-care advisors at the center of France's interwar commercial beauty culture sought to attract the practical woman of today by portraying beauty work as a scientific undertaking. Pursuing technological innovations in the manufacture and packaging of their aids, cosmetic firms offered safer, more effective products. Firms not only experimented with new ingredients; they also employed a form-follows-function aesthetic to craft eye-catching product packages, and they introduced novel product-delivery systems that accommodated the active woman's lifestyle. Beauty retailers, for their part, cultivated new relationships with female patrons. By envisioning women as informed purchasers who valued knowledge as well as results, retailers portrayed beauty work as a highly skilled, collaborative effort. In the women's press and in their self-care manuals, beauty advisors promoted a methodical, regimented approach to bodily maintenance. They offered women tips for streamlining their daily beauty routines, and they counseled them on how to choose and employ products. In these ways, they convinced "today's woman" that to take full advantage of the novel compacts, applicators, and systems at her disposal and to successfully cultivate a "healthy, natural beauty," she had to understand beauty as both a science and an art.

Examining precisely how manufacturers, retailers, and advisors appealed to woman's intellect as well as to her aesthetic sense, this chapter examines how the modern beauty industry developed in tandem with modern womanhood. Providing safe, competitively priced products that were multifunctional and decorative, firms adapted product fabrication and design. Equipping women with the latest products, confiding important beauty knowledge, and demonstrating the most up-to-date application methods, retailers and advisors provided women with the tools and strategies to make their own beauty. At the same time, women could not have *appeared* modern without the assistance of commercial beauty culture. Novel devices and time-saving techniques facilitated women's quotidian activities while colorful cosmetics enabled new forms of corporeal expression. Moreover, by depicting woman's pursuit of beauty as a reasoned but pleasurable personal undertaking, commercial beauty culture validated her desire to *be seen* as both smart and beautiful. Thus, at the intersection of culture and commerce, modern women and modern beauty made one another.

MANUFACTURING BEAUTY

The beneficiary of decades of industrial innovation, the vibrant commercial beauty culture that flourished in interwar France introduced consumers to an ever-widening array of cosmetic products and delivery systems. Experimenting with new, scientifically tested substances—synthetic as well as natural—firms expanded their product portfolios. Fabricating aids composed of safer ingredients that retained their hygienic properties and employing new materials to make product-delivery devices (applicators, containers, etc.) and packages, firms ensured product efficacy.[2] Through product fabrication and package design, interwar firms appealed to women who desired luxury but demanded functionality, who sought to live "honestly" but also "without any constraint."

Confronted with mounting competition from American companies and tasked with navigating a precarious global economic climate, the success of interwar French beauty firms was anything but a foregone conclusion. As consumer incomes became severely depressed and inflation rose to dramatic levels, American firms mass-produced and aggressively exported less expensive beauty products.[3] In magazine advertisements and on retailers' shelves, French consumers increasingly encountered Cutex nail enamels, Pond's creams, Pepsodent toothpastes, and Palmolive soaps.[4] Moreover, the influx of American-made products into the French market was accompanied by the establishment of American-owned firms within French cities. Dorothy Gray, Revlon, Harriet Hubbard Ayer, and Marie Earle all set up shop alongside Helena Rubinstein and Elizabeth Arden in the most desirable commercial neighborhoods of Paris.[5]

Despite these challenges, French firms like Chanel, Coty, and L'Oréal enjoyed tremendous success by expanding their operations and diversifying their product lines, measures that enabled them to increase revenues while making goods more accessible to a broader range of consumers. Following the lead of other prominent fashion designers who created perfumes and cosmetics to complement their fashion lines, Coco Chanel introduced her signature fragrance Chanel N° 5 in 1922. Along with business partners Pierre Wertheimer and Théophile Bader, Chanel founded Parfums Chanel, and in 1929, the company launched a global cosmetics line.

The same year that Chanel's prized fragrance reached the market, the esteemed perfumer François Coty launched his new perfume Paris, which became an instant best seller in England and America.[6] Paris marked the first of fifteen fragrances that Coty distributed internationally in the 1920s. Although the firm opened its New York subsidiary in 1912, it was not until after the war, when returning GIs brought Coty products home to their wives and girlfriends, that the brand resolutely established itself in the American market. Success in the United States, as well as the popularity of its fragrances at home, encouraged Coty to manufacture beauty aids in the postwar decade. Following industry trends, Coty introduced a variety of cosmetics aimed at enhancing woman's sex appeal. For example, other firms offered les Vampires eye shadow, poudre Nymphea, and poudre Mystérieux; even more eroticized, lipsticks carried names like le Caméléon and Délicia. Advertised explicitly as "pour le boudoir," Coty Fard Léger and its nail polishes, which were promoted as a "necessary part" of the "woman's seductive arsenal," explicitly evoked the sexual, while the firm's seemingly muted "rouge naturels" line included everything from subtle shades like "pale rose" and "invisible" to vibrant hues called "cherry" and "electric."[7] Through her use of lipsticks and nail polishes, today's woman, at least as Coty envisioned her, could play matron one moment and vixen the next.

Like Coty, L'Oréal had expanded its operations abroad in 1912. After the war, it distinguished itself by creating products suited to the popular bob hairstyle and to perms; however, the company also developed new lines of safe-to-use coloring products (Immédia, L'Oréal Simplex, L'Oréal Henné) that allowed women to change their look almost as frequently as they changed their clothing.[8] At the same time, L'Oréal began diversifying its product lines; purchasing the Monsavon soap company in 1928, manufacturing the first mass-marketed shampoo, DOP, in 1934, and introducing the first sunblock, Ambre Solaire, in 1935.[9] The firm even expanded its business repertoire, launching the lifestyle magazine *Votre beauté* in 1933 and sponsoring health and hygiene programs on French radio.[10] L'Oréal further increased its market base by targeting a growing group of beauty consumers: men. Firms had offered men shaving creams, hygiene products, colognes, and even hair dyes for decades; but in the 1920s, companies like Dorin introduced an entire line of beauty products for men, Dorin Pour Monsieur. The line included a *crème de toilette,* a loose powder, a portable pressed-powder compact, a *produit pour teinter,* and cream and powder antiseptic toothpastes. Meanwhile, L'Oréal postcard advertisements from the 1930s announced that the company's hair-coloring products were suitable for use by all members of the family, including "votre père." Through expansion and diversification, high-end firms like Chanel and Coty and companies like L'Oréal, which catered to a decidedly more modest clientele, survived the economic perils of the interwar years.

Firms further weathered the economic maelstrom by improving upon existing products, employing novel fabrication techniques that enabled quicker production and that ensured product consistency, and developing new goods to bring to market. Cognizant of the hazards associated with cosmetics use—the possibility of skin irritations and interactions, problems caused by inappropriate use, and the potential ills of applying substances to the skin that contained even trace amounts of lead, mercury, or arsenic—firms continued to pursue safer, less toxic ingredients. Synthetic components, in particular, made products last longer, made creams lighter, and made intense colors more transparent and less garish.[11] The integration of synthetic substances also permitted firms to experiment with color. Shades of mauve, blue, and green, which certainly required appropriate application so as not to make the wearer appear ghoulish, flourished alongside conventional browns, pinks, and reds. Innovations in the composition and fabrication of beauty aids also spawned the creation of entirely new kinds of products. Rice powders, rouges, and lipsticks increasingly competed for retail shelf space with liquid nail polishes, powdery blushes, mineral-based powders, and compressed compacts.

Firms eagerly broadcast the scientific merits of these ingredients, declaring that they ensured product efficacy while providing hygienic benefit. Helena Rubinstein's "skin food" and "pasteurized creams," for example, promised to nourish the skin, while Crème Activa argued that its products enabled women to completely "remove the mask of old age." Claiming that its creams were both laboratory-tested and "radioactive," Activa evoked science as a shorthand for quality.[12] The cleanser KEM-O-LITE, which was actually intended to "protect the skin," also displayed the word "radioactive" on its bar-soap packaging. It was promoted in the press as derived from a "boue volcanique naturelle" (natural volcanic mud), with the firm boasting its ability to convert volcanic mud into a safe but potent cleansing agent.[13] Interestingly, brands like Crème Activa and KEM-O-LITE seemed unconcerned that consumers might perceive something that was "radioactive" or composed of "natural volcanic mud" as possibly dangerous when applied to human skin.

Firms further expanded their offerings by manufacturing hygienic, unisex products like deodorants and toothpastes. Deodorants and antiperspirants (such as Odorono and Palmolive), promised to "prevent perspiration" in just two applications per week and permitted one to manage rather than merely mask body odor.[14] Short hair, which drew more attention to a woman's mouth and to her oral hygiene, necessitated the use of toothpastes, tooth creams, elixirs, and other antiseptics.[15] Le Dentol, which was not only "based on Pasteurian science" but also available in a variety of forms (liquid, paste, powder, and soap), competed on pharmacy shelves with the American import Pepsodent, which claimed to be created from the "most modern science of the art of dentistry," as well as with Bi-Oxyne, a two-in-one product that cleaned and "whitened teeth" while "destroy[ing] microbes" and "perfum[ing] the breath."[16]

Firms connected hygiene, beauty, and science in advertisements promoting both product necessity and ease of use.[17] Cédib claimed that "the science of beauty is enriched by a new creation le Renovateur Cedib." Intended to cover wrinkles, tone muscles, and regenerate facial tissues, this product should, its advertisements recommended, become part of every "elegant Parisienne's" toilette. A *Vogue* advertorial from 1936 featured six products, all of which were celebrated for their efficacy, adaptability, and ease of use. Cédib's twenty-minute home beauty mask, la Crème nutrive reconstituante, promised to rejuvenate the skin by tightening pores, toning muscles, and acting as an astringent. Applied either before or after physical activity, Glaciale Keva lotions enabled users to retain their freshness even through physical exertion. Klytia's powdery makeup, distinguished by its unique applicator, provided wearers a natural look unachievable with a conventional powder puff. Arden's lipstick compact, packaged in a variety of jewel tones, accentuated a woman's fashionable wardrobe. Finally, Prince Matchabelli's delicately scented perfume pledged to skillfully "penetrate" without overpowering the wearer's natural scent. *Vogue* reiterated what beauty firms had expressed for more than a decade: the first step to achieving beauty was choosing the right product. Effective beauty work, moreover, required knowledge—knowledge of ingredients, of application method, and of execution. In short, the beautiful woman was also, necessarily, a smart consumer.

Vivaudou creams, although advertised as cleansing products rather than antiwrinkle agents, relied on science, common sense, and scare tactics to attract potential consumers.[18] The 1924 advertisement for its Cleansing-Cream Carte Blanche offered women a synthetic remedy to the natural dilemma of aging.[19] The caption "Wilted at thirty" naturalized the aging process, as the word "wilted" explicitly connected woman to a fading flower. Despite conceding that aging is a natural process, the microscopic close-up of the woman's pores, along with text claiming that "in the midst of youth, so many women infect their skin with all types of creams containing poisons that settle in their pores," suggested that women were complicit in their physical deterioration. This woman is wilted at thirty, the advertisement implies, because she has injured her skin with harmful aids. Alas, the damage can be repaired and the youthful epidermis recovered if she "stops the massacre of her beauty before it is too late" and "begins today cleaning her face with Vivaudou's Cleansing-

Cream Carte Blanche."[20] Vivaudou would restore woman's natural youth and save her from the damage that she unknowingly inflicted upon herself.

L'Oréal conveyed similar messages in advertisements for its wildly popular hair dyes. These products were in such high demand, in fact, that a L'Oréal spokesman estimated that according to the number of boxes of hair dye sold to beauticians in 1931, L'Oréal would earn 300,000 francs for its coloring products that year alone. Moreover, the firm projected that its newest line, L'Oréal-Blanc, which was designed to even out salt-and-pepper tones, would attract three, four, or five hundred thousand new users in 1932.[21] Although both men and women purchased anti-aging products (especially hair dyes), ads for these aids frequently featured manufactured life experiences—romantic interludes, leisure activities, and social encounters—that targeted aging women. A 1922 ad for L'Oréal hair-coloring products, for instance, depicted a woman at a social engagement under the tag line, "The injustice of gray hair."[22] Completely ignored by the men congregated in the background, the woman is seated alone in the foreground, her hair completely hidden under a scarf. The text reveals that the "injustice" for this woman is that she has turned gray at the age of thirty-five. "Judged as too old" to "be asked to dance at the party," she is abandoned to "suffer the stigma of premature aging." Luckily, L'Oréal coloring products would ease her suffering and "restore the splendid color of youth."[23] Through the purchase and use of its products, L'Oréal pledged, woman could not only change her appearance but also improve her social life.

L'Oréal advertisements also connected women to the latest technologies through narratives of youthful liberation. In another solicitation for hair dye, L'Oréal's twenty-something female driver[24] connected youth with both unfettered sexual freedom and personal mobility. L'Oréal promoted the transformative and playful qualities of its coloring product by comparing it to the speeding car, whose movement is captured in the driver's dramatically blowing hair and scarf. The text celebrates youth: it claims that the "woman driver is astonishingly young" and refers to the car as a "toy." Both text and image emphasize the toy's promise of adventure as well as the woman's exhilaration as she "plays" with it. But there is more at stake here than mere play. The car also symbolizes speed, movement, and power; it embodies, as Wendy Parkins has claimed, the "quintessential modern experience—the fragmentation of perspective that exposes the fragility of subjectivity and the transience of beauty."[25] The ad's female driver is empowered; literally in the driver's seat, she is figuratively in control of choosing both her destiny and her destination. Thus L'Oréal's underlying message is that, like the car, L'Oréal hair-coloring kits positioned woman in the driver's seat, urging her to take hold of the transience of beauty and offering her the opportunity to choose either the well-traversed path to old age or the fast lane to eternal youth.

Firms also attracted consumers by designing clever product-delivery systems that facilitated efficient product use. In addition to manufacturing countless tubes, bottles, and jars specifically suited to woman's hectic lifestyle, they developed ingenious accessories and applicators (wands for mascara pots, compact eye shadow and rouge pots that fit discreetly within the palm of a woman's hand)[26] that made application easy. Targeting the "modern, active woman," the Kemolite salon presented its le Caméléon facial cream not in a conventional jar but in a small, sleek tube designed to be carried on one's person.[27] Although women could purchase Crème Simon in jar, bottle, and bar form, by 1925, they could also buy the popular product in a convenient tube.[28]

As with creams like Simon and le Caméléon, powder-delivery systems were increasingly sold in transportable containers. Bertimay offered loose powder in small sachets, while pressed powders became available in compact form.[29] Designed to be functional as well as fashionable, Lubin's Boite de Poudre & Fard (fig. 6.1) exemplified the technical ingenuity of interwar product packaging by providing two products in one.[30] Lubin's tiny, yet modish compact contained both a facial powder and a colored makeup to brighten cheeks or lips. Its small casing made it portable, while its smooth design appealed to the "elegant woman's" sense of polite decorum. The Nildé firm's two-in-one powder and rouge compact, proposed for evening outings, could be worn itself as a fashion accessory. Though slightly larger than the Lubin compact, the Nildé "boite-tamis inversable" proved equally discreet. The Sauzé company offered several two-in-one systems. Its compact, though offering only one cosmetic (powder), supplied an easy-to-use applicator and a "large mirror" for quick, circumspect touch-ups.[31] Additionally, the container promised to conserve powder freshness, to ensure against spillage, and to economize product use by "letting out only the amount that you need."[32] The firm's dual-purpose *rouge-estompe* offered this same convenience for lipstick. The lipstick tube, constructed to permit an "infinitely rational, practical manner of use," was composed of two elements, a replaceable cartridge to hold the pasty rouge and a spiral wand for easy application. The wand prevented residue from staining the user's hands while enabling her to spread the rouge

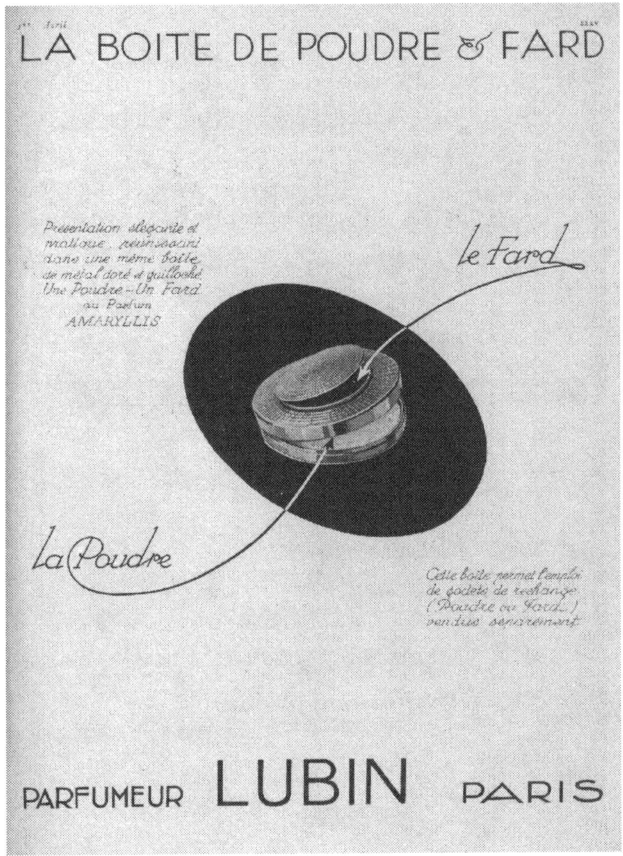

Fig. 6.1. Lubin's Boite de Poudre & Fard. *Vogue,* 1926.

evenly. The spill-proof cartridge, which held two different rouges simultaneously (one color for day and one for evening), was tightly packed to ensure that the product would not leak onto gloves or inside purses.

Improving on the two-in-one concept, firms began combining individual products into "kits" or "systems" so that consumers might address all of their skin-care needs with a single purchase. The extremely popular Vanity Kid line from the Marcel Franck firm combined powder, rouge, and perfume in stylishly decorated hand-held compacts. These kits, crafted to look like "modern jewelry," accentuated a woman's wardrobe at the same time that they fit discreetly in the palm of her hand. Known for stunning art deco design and high-quality craftsmanship, the Franck firm applied to its compact kits the same aesthetic sensibility it used to create its successful perfume atomizers. Square in shape, the Vanity Kid compact resembled a miniature camera, with two round cylinders on either end, one containing lipstick, the other perfume, and a circular compact containing compressed powder located at the center. Similar attention to detail characterized Dorin's beauty boxes. Sold in both cardboard and metal containers, Dorin's hand-held rouge and powder compacts opened like a tiny two-tier suitcase, revealing rouge and applicator on one level, and powder and application puff on the other. The small mirror inserted into the top of the compact provided a woman with all she needed to freshen up anywhere.

At the same time that firms adapted product design to the active woman's lifestyle, they created cosmetic packages that, like the new fashions, followed a modernist design aesthetic.[33] However, whereas fashion designers like Erté and Elsa Schiaparelli drew inspiration from the subjective and symbolic movements of cubism, surrealism, and futurism, cosmetic manufacturers incorporated purist and art deco elements.[34] Many firms blended these schools, combining the functional interests of purism (the singularity of form, the multiplicity of purpose, and the hybridization of object with subject) with the decorative, lavish flourishes of art deco, to transform compact cases, powder sachets, lipstick tubes, and rouge pots into incredibly functional, miniature works of art.[35] Firms were particularly attentive to the aesthetics of powder compacts. The poudreuse Sauzé that provided users with an easy-to-use application wand and serviceable mirror was also intentionally designed to double as jewelry.[36] Advertisements touted this feature as one of the product's premier advantages, claiming that "as a small piece of modern jewelry," the compact's "rare elegance" conveyed the "good taste" of the woman who used it.[37] Through the repetition of simple, symmetrical forms—a geometric crosshatch along the periphery of the compact lid encapsulates an equally simple, purely decorative interlaced flower pattern—and constructed not of traditional jewelry material (gold, silver, precious stones) but of cool, durable metal, the Sauzé compact exemplified modern, elegant design.

The same strategies used for compacts were also applied to other forms of cosmetic packaging. The clean lines and austere label of Chanel N° 5 perfume bottles and the sleek look of Antoine's cream astringent containers reflected a minimalist, form-follows-function aesthetic. Slightly more ornate than Chanel's and Antoine's bottles, Worth's containers for its Sans adieu line, which included perfume, powder compact, and lipstick, experimented with shape. Positioned on a two-tier square platform and topped with a spiral cylinder, the perfume container hardly resembled its Chanel rival, while the rectangular compact and lipstick tube contrasted starkly with the circular and round shapes favored by many competitors. Coty's new *rouge à lèvres automatique* also adopted the rectangular shape; however, when the tube was stood up on its base, it looked more like a tiny skyscraper than a modest beauty aid. Sporting thin, mathematically precise lines, symmetrical forms, and cast in gleaming metal, the Kadeko Derma skin-care line celebrated the artistry of the machine age by recalling the patina as well as the shape of an artillery shell.[38]

Firms assuaged the ordinary woman's desire for glamour not only through innovative design but also by hiring celebrities to endorse their products. While performers like Renée Deville endorsed Kijja's entire line of "Egyptian" cosmetics, Edmée Favart ("la grande artiste de l'Opréra-Comique," as she was identified in the ad) vouched only for Dorin's "Slip" hair-removal agent. Other firms employed several actresses at once. The Cadum Soap Company constructed dozens of advertisements that spotlighted the Guy Sisters; however, they also ran others featuring up to twenty-five performers at the same time. In an issue of *Vogue* from 1924, the company took out a full-page ad entitled "L'art et la beauté rendent homage au Savon Cadum."[39] The ad included miniature headshots of twenty-three actresses (and their autographs) organized around a mirror in the center filled with text that began, "The most beautiful and most celebrated artists of Paris attribute their beauty to Cadum Soap."[40] Encouraging readers to select the performer whom they regarded most attractive or with whom they most identified, Cadum acknowledged diversity among beauty ideals and beauty consumers.

The beauty industry's commitment to innovation was put on display at the Fourth French Exposition of Hairdressing and Perfumery in 1931. Essentially a national trade show where beauty professionals congregated to display their products and advertise their services, the expo reflected, in microcosm, fundamental transformations under way within French beauty business. The carnivalesque atmosphere of the event, made possible by colorful lighting and elaborate staging (techniques borrowed from both French department stores and American retail sites), demonstrated the industry's adoption of modern marketing techniques. Firms represented at the expo purchased booths to display their products, which, taken together, constructed a miniature city of beauty; an international emporia that, by exhibiting high-end products alongside discount brands, visually embodied the transition from a bourgeois to a mass consumer society.[41]

From their inception, expos were intended to enhance trade, promote new technologies, and invent new ways to stage manufactured objects.[42] Expos enjoyed a long and illustrious history in France: the government had funded display centers featuring industrial and craft produce since the reign of Louis XIV; the *expositions universelles* of 1889 and 1900 attracted international attention to French industrial and architectural ingenuity; and the 1923 Salon des art ménagers proved such a success that it reoccurred annually between 1926 and 1983.[43] Thus, by the time that cosmetic companies, perfumers, and hairdressers assembled in Paris in 1931, the trade expo was a well-established component of French industrial life.

The first three expos, held in 1922, 1924, and 1927, attracted a large number of exhibitors and patrons. *La coiffure de Paris,* which cosponsored the event with the Comité Marcel, noted a dramatic revenue increase from the first expo to the fourth. Revenues grew by 99,000 francs between the 1922 and the 1924 expo, and they jumped an astounding 643,000 francs between 1924 and 1927. As the French economy declined into depression in 1931, the journal estimated that the expo would take in 1.8 million francs (an increase of 892,000), almost doubling its earnings from 1927.[44]

The expo attracted a variety of participants and featured exhibits from an assorted collection of firms. One of the show's most striking features, in fact, involved the arrangement of exhibitor booths. Stands were erected in halls numbered 1 and 3. Hall number 2, which housed a runway, had been designated as the *salles de fêtes* and was the only room that did not include display booths.[45] Roughly equivalent in size, booths for elite perfume houses like Parfumerie Monpelas and L. T. Piver stood alongside or nearby booths devoted to less expensive brands like L'Oréal hair dye, Monsavon soap, and Odorono deodorant. Booths clearly reflected the character of the firm, its products, and its intended clientele. The Monsavon booth, for instance, complete with white porcelain sinks, tiled floor, and carefully arranged packages of soap, resembled a household bathroom and promoted a sterile, sex-neutral image of cleanliness that mirrored the purpose of its product. Conversely, the lavish Monpelas exhibit for its Malceïne cream, anchored by two huge sprays of fresh flowers and set up to feature the intricate design of its product packages, indulged the senses, conveying an image of luxury, good taste, and opulent femininity.

Erected as miniature boutiques representing a specific firm, exhibition booths reflected the French proclivity toward the retail site devoted entirely to one item. That exhibit booths were neither segregated by the price points of their wares nor differentiated by the amount of space allocated to their stands suggests that expo organizers regarded its participants as equal players on the field of beauty retail. The exhibition hall was, in this respect, a democratized space; by showcasing high-end beauty products alongside less expensive ones, the hall created the visual illusion of social leveling. In a business notorious for promoting market segmentation and for distinguishing elites from everyone else, the expo signified a rare moment of class mingling and interfirm collaboration. In this way, the Fourth French Exposition of Hairdressing and Perfumery exemplified the vibrancy of the interwar commercial beauty industry and blended a time-honored French tradition with a growing international impulse for mass consumption.

Within the context of a weakened interwar economy, the French luxury trades, of which the beauty industry comprised a notable segment, struggled to retain financial viability. However, for firms willing to innovate and to adapt—to research and employ new ingredients in product fabrication; to use unconventional materials in the construction of product applicators and containers; and to envision package designs that would appeal aesthetically and practically to consumers—beauty remained a feasible, even lucrative enterprise. By combining aesthetics with technology and portraying their wares as suitable for and suited to a certain kind of active, attractive, discerning woman, firms not only manufactured beauty products, but they also produced a new model of modern womanhood—the smart consumer. Appealing to the woman who desired to *be seen* as both intelligent and beautiful, firms provided the tools necessary for self-invention at the same time that they reinforced the notion that feminine identity was both performative and purchasable.

MARKETING BEAUTY

Beauty retailers, particularly beauty institutes, Prix Unique stores, pharmacies, and hairdressers solicited the savvy consumer by employing innovative marketing strategies. Playing equally on her pragmatism and her aesthetic sensibility, these retailers combined the science of selling with the art of display to transform their stores into modern, service-oriented enterprises. As the number of beauty institutes swelled in the interwar period, proprietors realized that they had to provide more than products and services to maintain their clientele. The most successful institutes attracted customers by selling experiences of glamour and respite as well as by imparting valuable beauty knowledge. The Prix Unique offered little in the way of luxury, but by selling serviceable products at low prices, it appealed to working-class women and to women who appreciated a good value. Characterized by well-organized shelves, brightly lit aisles, and seemingly endless selection, the discount store made beauty accessible to all. Smaller in size and stocked with fewer goods, the pharmacy continued to offer a wide range of health and beauty aids; to reach new customers, pharmacists attended to aesthetics and to functionality in their in-store displays. Finally, hairdressers parlayed the trust that they had established with long-term patrons with skill and kindness to retain customers. Acknowledging that their commercial success depended upon their ability to meet the demands of today's woman, interwar beauty retailers endeavored to become *bon commerçants.*

Providing beauty services and sharing coveted beauty knowledge, institutes played on woman's aesthetic sense as well as her practicality. Institutes trained and employed professional aestheticians who understood how to accentuate a woman's most attractive features. Individual consultations were rather pricey, as women could expect to pay fifty francs for a single consult in 1928. Yet for their investment they received elaborate facials, personal color consultations, and hair-removal treatments performed by skilled professionals.[46] Seriously engaged in scientific research and actively fabricating their own creams, serums, and cosmetics, institutes manufactured many of the products used and sold in their stores. By packaging their own multistep skincare systems—kits that could be used in the salon or purchased by patrons for home use—institutes made beautification accessible at the same time that they reinforced the idea that beauty was achieved only through product use, know-how, and personal commitment.

Promoting their skin-care systems as indispensible weapons in woman's chronic battle against old age and ugliness, institutes like Helena Rubinstein and Elizabeth Arden encouraged women to adopt a methodical, scientific approach to self-care. In a series of advertisements from *Vogue* in 1922, Rubinstein's products were touted as "tested by dermatologists throughout the world and trusted by . . . the prettiest women in society and on the stage."[47] Advertisements frequently encouraged consumers to come into the institute so that they could experience the "scientific treatment of the great artist."[48] Two years later, Arden's advertisements in *Vogue* lauded the "Méthode Scientifique, Elizabeth Arden" and invited potential customers to entrust themselves to "Elizabeth Arden[, who] employs the resources of science and art to perfect each detail of the face and body."[49] Patrons who could not visit the institute for a personal consult could beautify at home by purchasing products through the mail. In fact, both Rubinstein and Arden invited customers to call or write the facility for free brochures that detailed institute methods or to request personalized consultations by cutting out and sending in "diagnostic" questionnaires. By tailoring the three-step system to the individual, offering mail-order consults, and making beauty work easy to carry out at home, Rubinstein and Arden ensured that women could buy their products even if they never set foot in an institute.

Sporting names like Crème Pasteurisée and Évolution, several of Helena Rubinstein's product lines explicitly conjured scientific associations. The company announced its new line Évolution this way in *Vogue:* "Helena Rubinstein is launching a newly designed makeup this autumn because it is not pleasing enough to color one's face red or to over-embellish it with large quantities of powder. Makeup should, while being unobtrusive, give woman the sort of radiance that is noticed and admired." The result of many "long years of research," the Évolution line drew on "dermatological discoveries" to create an "entirely new formula" for its powder, lipstick pencil, and acidic cream makeup remover. Available in ten shades, the powder promised to "naturally" preserve the skin without clogging pores, while the cream astringent reinforced the skin's suppleness by simultaneously cleansing the epidermis and preventing wrinkles.

In addition to products boasting scientific value, the institute also offered treatments that promised the latest techniques to help woman preserve her youth. One of the more involved of these procedures was the Traitement Bio-Physique, a four-step process that relied on multiple techniques to "transform" and "renovate" a woman's face. The steps, each carried out by a trained aesthetician, included an unspecified mechanical procedure that purified the skin; a chemical treatment that would nourish and "naturally regenerate" the epidermis; the application of "electrical currents" intended to stimulate circulation; and finally, a cold radiation treatment that provided proper pore respiration. Aimed at the "woman who looked to science" for rejuvenation, this complicated procedure offered to restore youth using the most cutting-edge techniques.

Of course, institutes continued to appeal to woman's desire to appear young and sexy as well as clean. A 1922 advertisement for Phebel's anti-wrinkle clay mask played on these competing desires.[50] The tagline, "modern woman, modern care," runs parallel and diagonal to the image of a woman at her toilette, so as to draw the viewer's attention to the model's face. The woman removes the mask, which promises to "restore youth" and to eliminate "traces of a full day's fatigue," to reveal perfectly plucked eyebrows, pearly white teeth, and shimmering red lips. This process of self-revealing is both empowering and seductive: on the one hand, it liberates woman by erasing the signs of aging and encouraging her to take pleasure in self-care; on the other, the act of peeling away the mask mimics the act of disrobing, of exposing the intimate, the hidden, and the private to public view. The extent of woman's empowerment, however, is limited by the knowledge that to maintain her youth and beauty, she must wipe away one mask (the clay cleanser) only to recover her face with another (makeup). Nevertheless, by stripping away the metaphoric old mask, she succeeds in repairing her skin and creating herself anew.

A similar advertisement for a line of Helena Rubinstein makeup (fig. 6.2) explained the importance of selecting products that complemented the individual's wardrobe and that harmonized with her complexion. Fortunately, Helena Rubinstein, who has "devoted her entire life to feminine beauty," offers a matte cream rouge, a rouge compact in various shades, as well as two "refreshing" and "adherent" foundation powders and a lipstick that conveys the "clean and rich color of life."[51] The ad promises that these products would not only enliven the "dullest face" but also provide a "richness of color" that extends "charm and irresistible seduction to any woman."[52] The model's pouty lips, colored a deep red ("the allure of the rose") and the inviting slant of her chin and eyes challenge the viewer to "read" her body, while the curvy line that defines that body draws the viewer's eye to her embellished face. A silhouette only, the woman in the ad has no real body—she lacks substance. What matters, the ad implies, is on the surface only. The coquettish pose, the flirty tilt of the eyes, and a sensuous nonbody that acts as a human billboard for Rubinstein cosmetics coalesced to objectify and sexualize the female form. Thus this ad not only acknowledged the sexual play made possible by cosmetics, but it also demonstrated the symbiosis between a woman and her makeup to imply that each (woman and cosmetic, subject and object) spoke for the other.

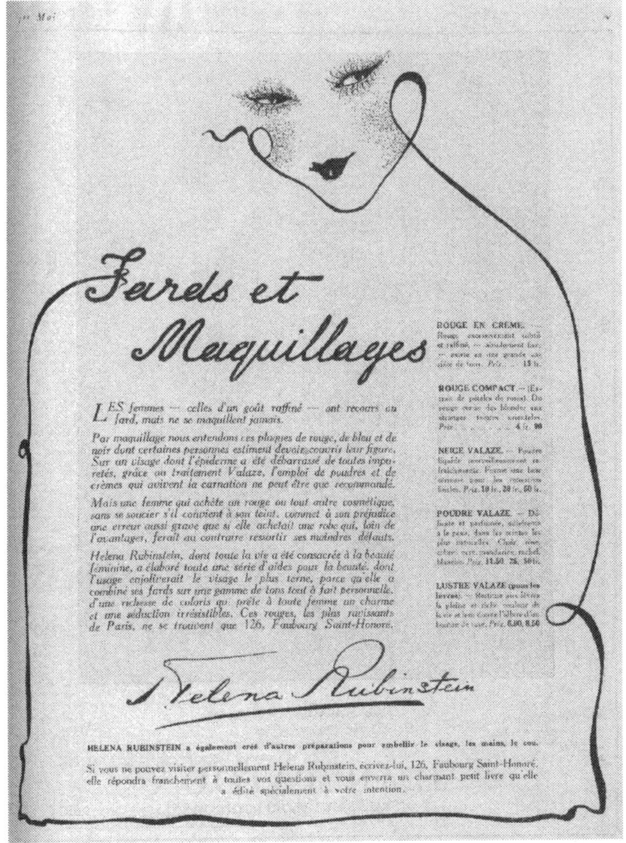

Fig. 6.2. Helena Rubinstein ad. *Vogue*, 1922.

Stylish institutes were not alone in endorsing scientifically tested products and advocating a systematic approach to beautification. In addition to typical products and services, clinics offered more invasive treatments, such as cosmetic surgery, tattooing, electrolysis, and *émaillage,* they employed licensed aestheticians, and they often staffed their facilities with certified health-care professionals. Training aestheticians to use "rational treatments with incomparable scientific products for the health and beauty of the face and body," and servicing a large clientele, the Keva Institute exemplified the thriving beauty clinic.[53] Keva resembled other institutes in that it sold wrinkle creams and eye makeup, provided facials and individual consultations, and circulated manuals containing tips from the clinic's "artistes."[54] Unlike other institutes, however, Keva also provided "aesthetic operations" conducted not by "artistes" but by a "specialist surgeon attached to the institute."[55]

Indeed, cosmetic surgery was an increasingly available option.[56] By the mid-1920s, doctors had performed hundreds of nose jobs, breast augmentations, and face-lifts.[57] To legitimize their aesthetic work, cosmetic surgeons argued that they provided a social and psychological service. By making men and women look younger, surgery, they argued, increased one's chances of obtaining employment and of attracting mates in a competitive marriage market. Dr. Suzanne Noël, a pioneer of aesthetic surgery and militant feminist, explicitly linked the new emphasis on appearance to the harsh times of the immediate postwar period when the struggle for existence was particularly precarious.[58] Moreover, surgeons equated ugliness with disease and maintained that unattractiveness caused psychological stress that was detrimental to both the individual and society.[59] In their efforts to legitimize aesthetic surgery, practitioners played on fears of aging, and even though many more women experimented with hair dyes and wrinkle creams than explored aesthetic surgery, the fact that these procedures were available indicated society's increased valuation of youthful beauty.

Despite their relative popularity, clinics came under attack for performing risky procedures. On June 6, 1926, the Superior Council of Hygiene published a brief article, "Institutes of Beauty Should Be under Surveillance," in which the author, who represented himself as a French physician, argued that all institutes needed regulation. Outraged by the number of patron injuries caused by the use of toxic ingredients, the improper application of products by institute staff, and the proliferation of "so-called doctors" (cosmetologists and beauticians who masqueraded as specialists "without a scientific degree"), the author demanded intervention. These charlatans who jeopardized the "health of women today," the author raged, "pose[d] a threat to the public health."[60] Whereas lifestyle journals like *Beauté* magazine praised the new clinics for offering sound advice and useful procedures, this author and others within the medical profession refused to recognize their scientific merit.

Debates about safe practices and practitioner qualifications aside, beauty institutes and clinics enjoyed tremendous commercial success. Patrons enthusiastically sought out professional treatments, relished the individual attention that they received from trained aestheticians, and purchased the products that they believed would make them beautiful. Selling experiences as well as products and services, moreover, institutes offered women a public space for creating new looks and performing new selves. But these experiences, procedures, and cosmetics came with such hefty price tags that institutes served a fairly exclusive clientele. Fortunately, the Prix Unique offered less affluent women access to quality beauty products at lower prices. Although not as glamorous as the institute and lacking a professional consultation, the Prix Unique nevertheless provided an array of beauty aids to women for whom beauty could only be achieved on a budget.

The Prix Unique brought less expensive, mass-produced beauty products to consumers with smaller discretionary incomes.[61] Modeled closely on Woolworth's American five-and-dime store (founded 1879), M. and Mme. Audibert's "one price" store Cinq et Dix opened in Paris in 1927. The success of Cinq et Dix encouraged several department store financiers to invest in the one-price business. In 1928, the Societé des nouvelles (along with a Hamburg department store consortium) founded Uniprix; Printemps opened Prisunic in 1931; and the Galeries Lafayette launched Monoprix (Rouen) in 1932. By 1935, France supported 166 Prix Unique establishments and about 30 of those operated within Paris.[62] Based on a sales philosophy of supplying quality products at an affordable price, the Prix Unique provided customers a no-frills, efficient shopping experience. Stores were systematically planned and organized so that not an inch of space went unused. Lighting, color, and music supplanted grand displays, elaborate *vitrines,* and prestige windows.[63] Items were meticulously arranged in glass cases, and the most frequently sought goods were located not at the back of the store but at the entrance. Every item sold at the Prix Unique was mass-produced, packaged for quick turnover, and intended to sell at the lowest market price. Even the process of selling was streamlined: prices were fixed and clearly exhibited, little money was allocated to advertising, and sales staff stocked shelves and doubled as cashiers.[64]

Goods for purchase generally belonged to one of three categories: convenience items, including food; shopping items like housewares, clothing and toiletries; and specialty items such as desk supplies and writing utensils.[65] Prix Unique stores offered personal-care items that were priced well below what pharmacies, salons, and élite institutes charged. Certainly, consumers could not purchase boutique brands at the one-price store. In fact, the Prix Unique intentionally eliminated all pretense of exclusivity for its products—a move that was potentially problematic for luxury items like cosmetics, whose cachet derived as much from their symbolic capital as from their utility. However, in the context of economic hard times, one-price stores provided serviceable toiletries at low prices. At the Prix Unique, consumers found a variety of shampoos, creams, soaps, deodorants, and toothpastes; and, as individual discounters began to expand, they also developed their own brands. In these ways, the Prix Unique brought beauty products to the masses.[66]

As the number of retail sites offering beauty products proliferated, retailers became increasingly attuned to using merchandising strategies that would give them a competitive advantage. Retailing trade journals, which employed a range of contributors from savvy publicity men to influential beauty industry leaders, urged French vendors to incorporate modern merchandising tactics and publicity schemes into normal business practices. French consumers were familiar with elaborate department store display windows, colorful periodical advertisements, and creative product positioning within shops. Yet, department store "prestige windows" that decorated the Parisian boulevard often did little to explicitly promote the objects for sale; periodical advertisements remained more developed and commonplace for some items than for others; and smaller shopkeepers frequently grouped products together illogically, in ways that maximized space but minimized visual appeal.[67] Trade journalists pushed pharmacists and hairdressers in particular to court the discriminating consumer by reimagining sales floors; more effectively displaying products in shop windows and on shelves; tailoring their business practices to consumer preferences; and taking better advantage of commercial advertising.

La publicité de France (1923–1947) offered merchandising and advertising advice for a variety of commercial enterprises; however, in 1923 and 1924, the journal dedicated a series of articles to one particular business: the pharmacy.[68] By the 1920s, not surprisingly, the neighborhood pharmacy was well established within cities and towns throughout the country. In 1923, A. Coulonge estimated that there was one pharmacy per 2,500 inhabitants in French cities and one per 4,640 inhabitants nationwide.[69] Pharmacists continued to be the primary retailers of medicines, but other pharmacy staples (specifically toiletries) were also sold in department stores, hair salons, Prix Uniques, and beauty institutes. Contributors to *La publicité de France* told pharmacists that to compete successfully with other retailers, each pharmacy should operate as a "small, distinguished shop."[70] Yet, in January 1924, Coulonge continued to lament the poor and disorganized appearances of many pharmacies. He was especially dissatisfied with what he considered confusing and uninspired in-store displays. Customers should find stores "clean and engaging," he wrote, and bottles and containers should be "harmoniously" arranged so as to "invite a sale."[71] Pharmacists should pay special attention to the *étalage* because this display not only "constitutes an excellent publicity medium" (attracting potential clients and enticing them to enter the shop) but also reflected the character of the store itself. In-store displays and shop windows, moreover, required "taste, reflection, method, and planning" if goods were to be showcased most effectively for sale.[72]

In May of the same year, the contributor R. Lieters responded to Coulonge's article, initially commending his insights but then pointing out the "special challenges" pharmacists encountered when attempting to display their wares.[73] Pharmacies were comparatively small shops that carried a wide array of disparate products; and unlike salons that might devote an entire display area to one hair product or a beauty institute that might feature one skin cream, pharmacies did not often carry a large volume of a single product. This meant that creating a "harmonious" in-store display could be quite expensive, if not impossible. Furthermore, because the size and shape of many flasks, containers, jars, and bottles made them difficult to arrange, it was not always feasible to construct a mixed *étalage*. Lieters argued that it was precisely because of issues like these that pharmacists needed to learn the "art" of display. He then provided readers with step-by-step instructions—using department store set-ups as his model—for how to inexpensively and effectively create a pharmacy window exhibit. He detailed the necessary materials (e.g., glass shelves, vases) in which pharmacists should invest, and he recommended regularly changing the display to maintain the interest of frequent passersby, whom retailers should always consider potential clients.[74]

Yet pharmacists were not the only retailers targeted in the trades; hairdressers, too, were pressed to update their display techniques, to advertise more effectively, and to see themselves as skilled artisans who worked in the service of the customer. *La coiffure de Paris* (1909–present), a journal aimed expressly at hairdressers and their suppliers, frequently addressed the fundamentals of publicity and salesmanship. In a September 1925 column devoted to "salon affairs," an unidentified author explained that publicity should account for 3–7 percent of a salon's annual expenditure.[75] Effective publicity, moreover, accomplished three objectives: it announced the business to potential clients; it indicated the type of salon (e.g., *salon des dames; salons mixtes*); and it drew attention to the quality of its services. In a group of articles published in 1927, Robert Sauleau explained that the successful *étalage* exhibited novel installations (complete with decorative cubes and attractive lighting) and incorporated elements that reflected both the store and its neighborhood.[76] Many proprietors resisted product displays, complaining that they undermined the salon's image. Sauleau countered these protests with a simple argument: if patrons did not know the availability and price of products for purchase, they would not buy them.[77] He assured coiffures that because creative displays would attract customer attention, they would both move merchandise and maintain the shop's integrity.

Sauleau's suggestions revealed a new stage in the relationship between hairdresser and patron in which the coiffure was attentive to customer desires, competed for her business, and sought her satisfaction.[78] The master stylist M. Arvet-Thouvet told fellow hairdressers in his article for the paper that once a client entered the salon, it was the proprietor's responsibility to present himself, in all ways, as a "bon commerçant."[79] A respected and well-known Parisian coiffure, Arvet-Thouvet had served as the secretary of the École supérieure de la coiffure, he was elected vice president of the Union Saint-Louis, and his shop at 335 rue Vaugirard serviced an international clientele.[80] He explained that hairdressers had to be the "artiste coiffeur" who devoted "body and soul" to his craft and to his staff as well as a "good" retailer who put the needs and desires of his customers above all else. To maintain a strong client base, he believed, the hairdresser had to satisfy every patron, treating each with kindness and patience.[81]

Achieving these goals meant catering to consumer demand. For example, hairdressers were also initially critical of the bob—not because of its social message but because they feared that women's haircuts would, like those for men, become too simple and low-priced.[82] Once hairdressers discovered that short cuts brought patrons into the salon on a more frequent basis and gave them more opportunity to sell clients other services (perms, manicures, and pedicures) and products (dyes, special occasion hairpieces, and cleansers), however, they, too, endorsed the new look. In their columns with such titles as "La manicurie," "La massage facial et les soins esthétiques," and "Les soins de beauté chez le coiffeur," contributors to the trade journal *La coiffure de Paris* energetically promoted the inclusion of new services.[83] They also advocated perfecting and diversifying traditional salon services, such as hair curling and hairpiece design. Perms and *postiches,* industry insiders argued, could feminize the masculine look and soften the features of the short-haired woman.

In addition to offering new services, hair-care professionals introduced a variety of new products intended to help women maintain the short hair-style. The celebrated Parisian hairdresser Antoine introduced a line of beauty aids under his name (fig. 6.3).[84] His cream astringent, for instance, promised to "nourish" the skin and to make the user's face, which the new hairstyle highlighted, clean and smooth. The product's function was then echoed in the sleek look of the astringent bottle itself, in its "clean" lines and "smooth" surface. The image of the attractive, well-coiffed model and Antoine's name displayed prominently on the cap proposed a luxurious and idealized image of modern femininity—an image that united beauty and hygiene in a youth-

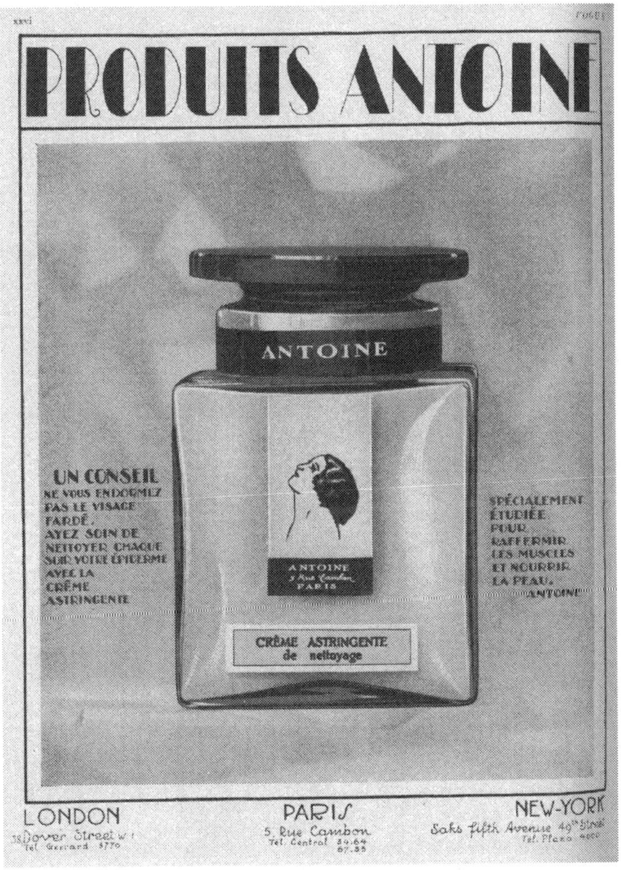

Fig. 6.3. Antoine Crème: Astringente de nettoyage. *Vogue*, 1927.

ful, stylish, nude female body. Other firms soon followed suit, responding to the fashion for short hair with cleansing agents, styling creams, treatments, and hair accessories that enabled women to achieve the desired style.

In the 1930s, hairdressers distinguished themselves from other beauty product retailers and service providers precisely through offering products consumers demanded and cultivating a relationship with salon patrons.[85] In contrast to businesslike pharmacists or *grand magasin* salesclerks who waited on dozens of anonymous shoppers every day, beauticians knew their customers intimately.[86] The coiffure was the client's friend, a person in her confidence, and someone who understood her individual desires.[87] Personal knowledge of one's patrons advantaged the hairdresser over other retailers because, as M. de Presle explained, "a woman who allows you to do her hair will seek your advice about makeup and perfume."[88] Thus the well-informed, retail-savvy hairdresser could build loyalty by using his or her intimate knowledge of the customer to guide her to the most suitable products.[89]

By the end of the decade, contributors implored hairdressers to increase their stake in the beauty business. The art of selling is "totally different" from the art of hairdressing or manicure, Gabriel Fau instructed readers in 1936. A customer will purchase beauty products in salons only if she is satisfied with the work performed on her hair. Therefore, Fau reasoned, hairdressers needed to know products and their applications so as not to lose client trust.[90] Additionally, products needed to be staged in such a way as to capture consumer attention and sensibly sorted so as to "create an atmosphere."[91] In 1938, an anonymously authored article questioned why salons were not yet major beauty product vendors. Uncertain as to the answer, the author emphasized that to compete with big stores salons had to attain customer satisfaction and stock quality products. This author also reiterated the points made by Fau and Arvet-Thouvet that coiffures needed to know their products, tailor stock to client needs, and use publicity wisely.[92] To make it in the increasingly competitive world of beauty sales, *La coiffure de Paris* contributors intimated, the hairdresser, like the pharmacist, had to reinvent himself as the *bon commerçant.*

Interwar beauty retailers engineered a variety of innovative marketing strategies. Attentive to the needs of the individual patron, beauty institutes, clinics, and salons provided a broad spectrum of services and a wide variety of products. The Prix Unique enlarged the consumer market for beauty products by offering buyers with limited budgets quality products at low prices, while the pharmacy became more attuned to the art of display, learning that the first step to making a sale was attracting attention. By redesigning displays, arranging products effectively, and reconceptualizing the relationship between vendors and customers, retailers acknowledged and reinforced the notion that as an informed consumer, today's woman valued both aesthetics and practicality.

MANAGING BEAUTY

In their beautification manuals and in their contributions to women's lifestyle magazines, interwar beauty counselors, like firms and retailers, promoted self-care as a serious, scientific undertaking. To this end, they advised women to streamline their beautification routines and to more efficiently manage their toilette. They reasoned that by judiciously purchasing and effectively employing commercial beauty aids—which should be regarded as essential components of every woman's beauty regimen—women could achieve expert results without completely emptying their pocketbooks. Advocating beauty work as a safe, scientific, and economical endeavor, advisors candidly appealed to woman's desire to *be seen* as both smart and beautiful.

Despite advice offered in magazines like *Femina* and *Vogue,* some women continued to obtain their beauty advice from lengthy manuals. Compared to the relatively short advice columns found in women's journals, interwar manuals, though fewer in number than their fin-de-siècle counterparts, remained popular among consumers and health-care professionals. Curtin's pocket-sized *Jeunesse et beauté. Vitalité. Ce qui l'augmente. Ce qui la diminue* appeared in its second edition in 1921, Courmont's seven-hundred-page clinical *Précis d'hygiène* was in its third edition by 1925, and a variety of other manuals were issued and reissued throughout the 1920s and 1930s. Interwar manuals, moreover, provided the same comprehensive coverage and detailed instruction as their prewar predecessors, but they promoted an even more streamlined approach to bodily care. The new generation of advisors who authored these manuals understood that, unlike the nineteenth-century woman who could devote an entire morning to her toilette, the twentieth-century woman's time was both limited and valuable. Manuals endeavored to make self-care less cumbersome and time-consuming; however, their very breadth and the lengthy set of expectations that they placed upon women often made conducting beauty work more rather than less burdensome.

Madeleine Ray's 1932 guide *Notre santé et notre charme* exemplified the trend among interwar manuals to endorse streamlined beauty routines. The guide followed the genre's conventional formula of organizing chapters thematically around specific areas of the body—chapter 4, for instance, was devoted entirely to the face.[93] Like her predecessors, she reiterated the belief that it was woman's responsibility to be beautiful and to teach cleanliness to her children. Even while relating the complex intricacies of the toilette, she insisted on a functional approach to self-care, explaining, as her predecessors had, the importance of a "hygienic" and "practically" arranged *cabinet de toilette.*[94] Ray's manual differed from its forerunners, however, in its advocacy of modern technologies (i.e., the home shower as useful for hydrotherapy treatments) and in its call for corporeal regimentation. Her book explored beautification procedures for the entire body and covered a range of diverse topics including oral hygiene, eye maintenance, hair care, body-odor management, and cosmetic application. Although she believed that fresh air and eating well were more beneficial to the complexion than cosmetics, rather than debate their utility (as earlier advisors had) she showed how strategically applied, high-quality aids could embellish and preserve woman's beauty.[95] Ray addressed each part of the body at length, accompanying her discussion of the need for cleanliness with precise step-by-step product-application plans. Take, for example, her instructions for "making a face," which involved the following five-step program: (1) choose and apply a good cream beneath a layer of rice powder; (2) apply rouge (in powder form) to cheeks, adding a little to the chin and earlobes; (3) apply a second coat of powder; (4) color eyelashes, brows, and lids with tints that match the eyes; and (5) apply lipstick by forming the mouth as though pronouncing the letter "i" during application.[96] A woman's face, Ray concluded, should form a perfect "V" shape and connote a scientifically organized, harmonious assembly of color and contrast.

Parisian hairdresser–turned–beauty institute proprietor Alfred Bitterlin took the scientific approach to beautification even further in his series of popular guides. Bitterlin used techniques learned while working alongside Mme. Le Brun at her institute. He communicated these techniques in two 1925 guides, *L'art du maquillage,* which sold for twenty francs and included eighty illustrations and sixteen color plates, and the more comprehensive but similarly priced *L'art de faire sa beauté.* In the introduction to the latter guide, Bitterlin explained:"I propose in this book to give you precious advice that I have acquired through experience and practice, on how to 'make your beauty.' It is an art to 'make your beauty' because every face offers originality, a personality, a 'type' that must be closely studied to be known."[97] Bitterlin regarded cosmetics as "tools that create the illusion of perfection"—tools that required skillful mastery before implementation.[98] Making up, he believed, was a "rational and scientific" process derived from a constellation of interrelated knowledge: women should "study" and "know" their skin types; they should account for the "play of light" against their skin and then select quality products suited to the time of day before following his "scientific method" to beautification.[99] Characterizing his prescribed routine as both suitable for "every skin type" and "impossible to mess up," Bitterlin explained that by paying careful attention to each part of the face, every woman could achieve "the illusion of true beauty."[100]

Creating the "illusion of true beauty," however, required that women choose suitable products and that they learn appropriate application procedures. Ironically, in the age of simplified fashions and easy-to-manage short hairstyles, new beautification practices necessitated that women devote more rather than less time to personal care. Take, for example, Sylvie's guide *Comment je fais ma beauté,* which supplied a simple chart for determining exactly how to carry out a regimen.[101] Sylvie's convenient table matched skin tones and hair colors to complementary shades of powder, lipstick, rouge, and eye shadow. It illustrated which hues were best suited to individual cosmetic users and also suggested how to harmonize different color combinations. Although the chart was intended to assist users by streamlining the process of making up, by emphasizing the seemingly infinite variety of possible combinations and demanding that the user match her skin tone and hair color to both the occasion and the makeup color, she demonstrated how the regimented approach to bodily administration complicated rather than simplified woman's beauty routine.

Glossy magazines offered a welcome alternative to lengthy, expensive manuals, especially for women who had neither the time nor the money to invest in complicated beauty regimens. Mimicking manuals, magazine articles began featuring at-a-glance charts, offering step-by-step application instructions, and providing pictorial illustrations demonstrating useful techniques. These tip sheets taught women how to employ vibrant colors and how to take full advantage of the new products coming to market. Yet rather than include these tools in bound, multichapter tomes, magazines supplied them in brief one- to four-page inserts that could be easily cut out for future reference. By including scientific advice and miniature manuals, moreover, magazines also advanced a rational approach to corporeal maintenance.

Although generally more attuned to aesthetics than to functionality, both *Femina* and *Vogue* published articles dedicated to the scientific aspects of beautification. In its autumn 1931 issue, *Femina* included the article "The Clarity of a Beautiful Face," in which the frequent contributor Françose Arnoux relayed Dr. Smol's research-based beauty advice.[102] A few months later, in February 1932, the magazine interviewed makeup artist Mme. Charol. In "The Science of Chemistry in the Service of Beauty," Mme. Charol explained how her scientific research on cosmetics in antiquity informed her work on current clients.[103] *Vogue* offered similar articles. As early as 1923, its piece "How to Conquer a New Youthfulness" argued that "today's fountain of youth" entails mechanics, chemistry, and electricity.[104] Evoking the utility of science and the merits of scholarly research articles like these revealed the extent to which *Femina* and *Vogue* acknowledged women's growing desire for practical, accurate information.

Magazines also began including miniature beauty guides within their monthly issues that, once extracted, could be used for daily consultation. In November 1932, for example, *Femina* included Marie-Claire Duchenne's "The Science of Beauty: Enriched Each Day by New Discoveries."[105] Conspicuously divided into five sections—(1) Physics and Chemistry Find New Substances; (2) Cleanliness and Coquetry; (3) Importance of the Beauty Institute; (4) Individual Makeup; and (5) Beauty Is Multiple and Diverse—Duchenne's ambitious guide covered in two pages what took authors of beauty manuals hundreds of pages to relay. Two years later, the magazine included a similar manual by Claude Malays, who published beauty and self-care articles every month in the magazine. In her "Petit bréviaire de la beauté," Malays promised to assist women in the daily beauty regimen by elaborating the thirteen steps needed to achieve a toilette that would "make them beautiful."[106] Along with her detailed instructions, she provided ten images illustrating the correct way to carry out her proposed routine.

Following the lead of successful magazines like *Femina* and *Vogue,* Eugene Schueller's *Votre beauté* offered women beauty advice, advertised the latest products and procedures, and instructed women in application techniques. However, *Votre beauté,* which had grown out of the trade journal *Coiffure de Paris,* proved, unsurprisingly, much more attuned to consumer desires. From its inception as a lifestyle magazine, *Votre beauté* addressed a broad, mixed-class audience and worked assiduously to incorporate reader concerns. Furthermore, the monthly encouraged reader feedback, soliciting and publishing hundreds of letters in the interwar period. Thus when *Votre beauté* advanced a scientific approach to self-care, it did so in response to reader demands, suggesting that pervasive discourses about streamlining and rationalizing the beauty routine not only reflected the agendas of beauty experts but also resonated with ordinary women who demanded tips on how to more effectively perform beauty work.

Responding to reader demand for more in-depth coverage of beauty product application, *Votre beauté*'s "Know Your Evening Makeup" article from its 1936 Christmas issue provided a "tracking table" intended to help women match their makeup to their hair color. Comprised of six rows (each row devoted to a specific hair color) and four columns of corresponding makeup options, the table offered readers a tool for discovering the "colors of blushes and powders suitable to your type." The undisclosed author of the article acknowledged that though it was "impossible" to please all readers, the goal of the chart was to "offer some general principles" that readers would find useful.[107]

In his October 1937 article "Individual Makeup: How to Create Your Own without Error," the contributor Michel Arbaud reiterated the notion that no single makeup suited every woman.[108] Despite the popularity of charts and tables intended to guide women in their beautification efforts, Arbaud cautioned that, "there can be no standard makeup." Rather than admire and attempt to emulate the makeup worn by friends, passersby, or celebrities, women should understand that "there is a different makeup for every woman." Indeed, he explained, "your makeup is one that makes 'you' more beautiful and that will enhance the character of 'your' face." Each woman, therefore, needed to "take into account two essential points when modifying her face, shape and color."[109] Once woman understood the shape of her face, her mouth, her eyes, and her nose, she could, Arbaud maintained, learn to create her "individual beauty." To guide women through this process, Arbaud included photos of five women with different hair and skin types positioned alongside drawings of these same women wearing makeup that produced different looks. He also offered two detailed tables as legends for the drawings to explicate how hair color could be matched with foundation, rouge, lipstick, and eye makeup. "Consulting these two tables, you will find not the final colors to make your ideal," Arbaud confessed, "but at least, a starting point that will allow you to avoid serious errors."[110] In a matter-of-fact tone and straight to the point, Arbaud implored women to consider their cosmetic choices carefully. He asked them to study their faces, their products, and their application methods—in short, to know the tools of beauty as well as they knew themselves.

An article that appeared the following month, "Knowing 'One's' Makeup Is Not Enough; We Must Learn to Execute," elaborated Arbaud's advice.[111] "In the October issue," the piece began, "we provided a convenient way to find the shape and color of makeup that could give your face the greatest value. But this is not all that you need to know. You still need to know how to apply makeup and perfume so that they perform their function adequately. . . . Here is a new process that will create the desired effect."[112] Drawing on new techniques used in Hollywood and in Parisian institutes, the authors recommended application procedures based on skin type (dry, oily, normal). The authors privileged skin type because, they argued, everyone's goal was to have beautiful skin, and knowing whether one's skin was dry or oily was the first step to realizing which products would provide a "natural" look. Giving the skin "color and texture," however, took both time and knowledge. Just as the application of products like rouge and powder should not be hastily applied, using ill-suited products should also be avoided. Providing photographic demonstrations and a twelve-step process for sectioning and tending the face, the article concluded with useful regimens for each skin type.

Attentive to the needs and concerns of its subscribers, *Votre beauté* published scores of letters from readers who sought advice about how to reduce the appearance of wrinkles, lose weight, or apply makeup.[113] Amid these requests were inquiries regarding less expensive beauty treatments. In response, the magazine published its lengthy article "Beauty Budgets" in April 1936. Authors engaged rudimentary market research practices by interviewing readers with a standard questionnaire about their quotidian beauty practices. Participants responded to three questions: (1) How much do you spend in one year to maintain your beauty? (2) What products do you need? and (3) How often do you go to the hairdresser? Most of the published responses came from readers who the magazine identified as "modest spenders." The first interviewee, for example, an unmarried secretary identified as blond and athletic with an annual income of 14,000 francs, confessed to spending 750 francs per year on self-care. She visited the hairdresser once a month, spent 40 francs a year on her nails, and purchased rouge, foundation, powder, and eye makeup as needed. Other women reported similar spending habits and confided that they used a combination of expensive (Lubin, Payot, Patou) and discount (DOP, Crème Simon) brands. One interviewee even admitted to buying ingredients from the pharmacy to mix her own products.[114] These responses reveal that women neither were loyal only to one brand nor did they purchase all their beauty products from the same retailer. Rather, they supplemented their high-end repertoire with discount brands, suggesting that they prized both efficacy and value.[115] Interested in women's purchasing habits as well as their beauty practices, *Votre beauté* validated woman's practical pursuit of beauty.

In their advice manuals and in their contributions to women's magazines, advisors coupled time-saving tips and shortcuts with practical suggestions for simplifying beauty routines. Whereas manual authors continued to provide painstakingly specific discussions of head-to-toe bodily care, magazine contributors concentrated their advice primarily on one area of the body (the face, the nails, or hair). Both manuals and magazines, however, advocated a regimented approach to bodily administration that was intended to streamline processes of beautification. Ultimately, by advocating economical, methodical approaches to beauty management, interwar advisors reinforced the prevailing sentiment among beauty professionals that modern women desired to *be seen* as both smart and beautiful.

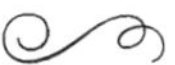

In the context of France's interwar commercial beauty culture, the process of making beauty modern was intimately and inextricably linked to the making of modern womanhood. Firms claimed to offer commodities that were effective (hygienic, safe, and developed through cutting-edge scientific research) and efficient (portable, decorative without ostentation, and easy to use); they used scientific ingredients; provided technologically advanced applicators and product-delivery systems; and streamlined package design in an effort to fit into the modern woman's busy life. In these ways, firms validated woman's pursuit of beauty and normalized her reliance on visible cosmetics. Beauty retailers began to envision modern women as discerning consumers who, neither motivated by conspicuous purchasing nor manipulated into indiscriminate spending, needed to be convinced as well as courted. Institutes, Prix Uniques, pharmacies, and salons sold experiences and imparted knowledge, while beauty counselors promoted a rational approach to bodily care.

In these ways, commercial beauty culture provided modern women with the tools and strategies necessary to make themselves visible, to shape how they viewed themselves and, to some extent, how they were seen by others. Moreover, it was precisely this new way of seeing the female self and the female body that marked today's woman as "completely different from women of the past." Yet, woman's relationship to beauty remained fraught with contradiction. The same cosmetics firms that fueled women's fantasies of eternal youth, promising them health and an antidote to the ravages of time, also expected them to commit to expensive, time-consuming beauty regimens. Ironically, however, even as beauty work exposed the theatrics involved in creating, maintaining, and performing the female self, cosmetic advertisements and beauty experts also pointed out the limitations of that liberation. As advertisements for wrinkle creams and hair dyes attested, woman may have been in the driver's seat, but she was also perceived as someone who needed to be rescued from social isolation and saved from her own self-indulgent narcissism. If woman wanted "to be seen" as powerful, sexy, young, and free, she had to purchase her "look" at the high price of dependence upon artificial creams and synthetic dyes.

The notion that the self was something to perform put such a premium on appearance and visibility that it threatened to place woman back into the role of the object on view. Moreover, women sometimes forfeited individuality to a homogeneous and homogenizing fashion ideal by aspiring to achieve "a look." In his documentary concerning France's interwar beauty industry, Louis Léon-Martin offered this impression of women leaving a Parisian beauty institute. "As the women exit, their faces are identical: the same pencil line at the bottom of the brow, the same brown eyelids, the same black lashes, even the lipstick, the same pink temples, the same white nose tip.... Apart from age or dimensions, they all look alike," he explained. "The house provides universal beauty, unique and egalitarian. Beauty is not a question of character; it is a question of caliber. There is a standard type created through concentrated Taylorized services.... Twenty times I see the same face and the same silhouettes pass by."[116]

CONCLUSION

In the spring of 1949, the Commission intersyndicale de la parfumerie conducted an "Étude du marche de la parfumerie."[1] Although the stated aim of the project was to ascertain the "general opinion of women regarding the use of perfumery products,"[2] the investigation surveyed 600 men in addition to 8,400 women. The study attempted to assess consumer attitudes and to determine spending patterns as they pertained to perfume, *eau de toilette,* hair-care agents, and other beauty products. Investigators canvassed the country and interviewed 1,350 women from each of five regions (North and East; West; Center; Southwest; and Southeast). Researchers not only subdivided interviewees according to geography (region and number of inhabitants per city) but also grouped them by social class, age, and marital status.

Investigators presented their results in the form of rudimentary shaded boxes, charts, and graphs that indicated consumer responses to individual questions. For example, interviewers asked, "Do you consider beauty product usage a luxury or a necessity?" Sixty percent of all interviewees responded that it was a necessity. Statistics showed that women with higher incomes were more likely to hold this view than women with lower incomes; that women under the age of thirty-five (women born after the Great War) were more likely to regard beauty-product use as necessary than were women thirty-six and over; and that single women and married women were equally as likely to consider it necessary.[3] The study also presented data for specific types of products: 75 percent of interviewees acknowledged that they regularly used face powder; 70 percent that they wore lipstick; 60 percent that they applied beauty creams; 23 percent that they polished their nails; 13 percent that they used eyeliner, and so on. In their responses, interviewees confided their personal hygiene and beauty habits; revealed where and how they shopped for beauty aids; shared their beauty budgets; and pointed out the types of publicity that they considered most persuasive.

Studies like this one do more than simply attest to the success of France's commercial beauty culture in the mid-twentieth century; they also demonstrate an evolution in French attitudes toward artificial embellishment. On a basic level, the study assumes the social acceptance of beauty products among consumers. Like Colette, they assumed that makeup had become "as ordinary as food." Indeed, the notion that French women regularly used cosmetics was old news by 1949. In addition to booming sales figures and the continued proliferation of manuals and lifestyle magazines devoted to beauty, women's memoirs from the interwar period attested to the important role cosmetics played in women's lives. As early as 1920, Liane de Pougy claimed that "nowadays there are a lot of pretty girls[;] cosmetics diminish the gap between beauty and mediocrity."[4] Makeup had become so essential to the wealthy literary bohemian Clara Malraux that she took it with her on her long journeys to the most remote villages of Indochina. Knowing the value of her stock, she admitted that she was careful to "be economical with what lipstick I had: it was still Guerlain's."[5]

By focusing on female consumers specifically, the investigation legitimized woman's reliance on commercial beauty aids and her participation in consumer society at the same time that it highlighted the myriad ways that beauty and femininity remained inextricably linked. The six hundred men included in the interview were issued a special questionnaire, asked only about hair products, and relegated to one chapter. Women occupied the other seven chapters, and it was women who were asked about their habits, their preferences, and their practices. The study thus implied that if beauty had evolved from a luxury into a necessity, if it was practiced by the affluent as well as the financially challenged, by the youthful as well as by the aging, by Parisienne as well as by *paysanne,* it remained nevertheless woman's responsibility.[6]

Throughout this book, I have argued that beauty figured prominently in French assumptions about womanhood. In the early nineteenth century, feminine beauty was both considered natural and naturalized within scientific, political, and philosophical discourses. Significantly, the expectations placed upon women by statesmen, health-care professionals, and even cultural elites were rooted in theories of biological sex difference. In the main, beauty was not only regarded as an essential component of femininity but also circumscribed as a female duty. As concerns about personal hygiene and public health increased toward the end of the century, women became responsible for ensuring individual, familial, and national cleanliness.[7] Indeed, it became as much a woman's duty to produce healthy bodies for the nation as it had always been her responsibility to effectively reproduce its citizens. One consequence of this imperative involved a shift in attitudes concerning commercially fabricated beauty products. Beauty aids, especially cleansers, were no longer ridiculed as immoral agents of depravity but were now mobilized as salubrious soldiers in the war against germs, disease, and depopulation. In this way, beauty work, as a necessary companion to hygienic bodily care, became a mechanism for ensuring nothing less than the survival of the French race.

From the late nineteenth century onward, the products, institutions, and discourses of France's commercial beauty culture played an increasingly important role in producing the feminine. Alongside cosmetics and perfumery firms, coiffeurs, pharmacists, and self-proclaimed beauty experts saturated the market with a variety of new synthetic cosmetic products: creams, dyes, kohls, and powders. Women also learned about these new products through a vibrant and diverse set of commercial discourses, advertisements and fashion magazines chief among them. Meanwhile, they learned how to care for their bodies in salons, cosmetology schools, and beauty institutes. At the fin de siècle, commercial beauty culture not only introduced middle-class French women to an array of personal-care products, but it also taught them how to use these products effectively and with discretion.

By the early twentieth century, appearance was becoming more than merely a marker of class or gender; it became, in fact, a production and a "constituting act."[8] Beauty played an integral role in woman's self-production. In the theater, in her fiction, and in her real life, Colette evoked beauty to embody and to propagate multiple versions of womanhood. In the interwar period, beauty became constitutive of womanhood in new ways, serving as a medium for self-expression and as an acknowledged line of demarcation between self and other. Although she was highly critical of fashion and cosmetics, even Simone de Beauvoir admitted that "techniques of appearing"[9] had gained in importance among French women precisely "because in illusion it [the toilette] enables them to remold the outer world and their inner selves simultaneously."[10] Whether considered a natural aspect of woman's sex, a respectable woman's responsibility, or a tool in the act of self-creation, beauty not only marked French women; it also functioned as a critical register through which the feminine was produced.

A second argument of this book has been that the institutions, discourses, and products of France's commercial beauty culture operated simultaneously as sites of gender construction and contestation. On the one hand, conventional notions of beauty were evoked to legitimize woman's subordinate status and to qualify other arbitrary characteristics ascribed to her sex. On the other hand, women employed beauty to challenge these assumptions, to take possession of their bodies, and to perform new identities. When conceptualized as a natural sex characteristic, beauty supported the myth of the eternal feminine—a myth that eschewed human agency and portrayed gender identity as something fixed and stable. However, when conceptualized as a form of work, a production, or an illusion, beauty exposed gender as a performance.

Gender as performance fundamentally changes how we regard the relationship between women and beauty. Gender performativity, as Judith Butler argues, opens a space for subversion by calling attention to how "an identity is instituted through a *stylized repetition of acts.*"[11] One way that *The Force of Beauty* has explored this idea is by analyzing how women were constructed as decorative objects. Upheld as the "fairer sex," women were characterized as naturally inclined toward adornment and innately interested in physical appearance. Throughout the nineteenth century, middle-class women reinforced this idea by indulging in *maquillage invisible,* by keeping up on the latest trends, and by perfecting their personal toilette. However, fulfilling the role of decorative object not only reinforced gender norms; it also became a way to challenge them. The heroines in Colette's novels, for example, embraced woman's object status. Renée and Léa, the actress and the courtesan, lived on the social fringe, were sex objects, and were completely aware of themselves as performers. Although cosmetics provided these women a form of packaging and represented the complete commodification of the female body, Colette suggests that by self-consciously embodying the decorative object, by performing the self as decorative object, Renée and Léa challenged the notion of identity fixity. Significantly, beauty was central to each heroine's identity performance, and with each pat of the powder puff and each swipe of the mascara wand, these characters revealed beauty as a choice rather than a destiny.

In the interwar period, commercial beauty culture enabled women from all backgrounds to create and perform new identities. Women used cosmetics to embody a range of identities, from the androgynous *garçonne* to the hypersexualized femme fatale. They were inspired by women on the boulevard, by women on posters and in magazines, and by women in the cinema. Importantly, the beauty industry itself recognized financial opportunity in woman's desire to experiment with her image. Firms offered a battery of new products, aggressively advertised in the media, and even sponsored contests. Commercial beauty culture multiplied the possibilities for woman's self-expression; however, lurking in the shadows of these performances was the unsettling possibility that female identity might be reduced entirely to appearance. Gender as performance might destabilize and denaturalize gender categories, but it might also prevent woman from creating an authentic self.

In the post–World War II period, Simone de Beauvoir was very much aware of the problems that women encountered when they engaged in these precarious performances. She viewed fashions and cosmetics as nothing more than props that reinforced woman's subordinate status. "It is not only that girdle, brassiere, hair-dye, and make-up, disguise body and face," she wrote, "but that the least sophisticated of women, once she is 'dressed,' does not present *herself* to observation; she is, like the picture or statue, or the actor on the stage, an agent through whom is suggested someone not there—that is, the character that she represents but is not."[12] Beauvoir argued that gender performance does not liberate woman but rather reimplicates her in the very system that she has sought to transcend. For her, natural or artificial, beauty does little else than continuously re-produce woman as the second sex.

Perhaps this last point helps explain why twentieth-century feminists and scholars of women's history have been so reluctant to take beauty seriously as a constitutive element of feminine identity. During the women's liberation movement, it was commonplace to represent the beauty and fashion industries as patriarchal, capitalist oppressors and to regard the women who participated in beauty culture as misguided or manipulated.[13] By focusing on the complicated and sometimes symbiotic relationship between women and commercial beauty culture, I have explored how and why beauty posed contradictions for French women during the Third Republic. Evoked in support of the eternal feminine and prescribed as a social duty, beauty has discursively positioned woman within a constraining set of interlocking assumptions that have limited her socially, economically, and politically. But beauty has also served as a vehicle of self-expression, and it has empowered women to challenge convention. In these years, as beauty products evolved from luxuries into necessities and as women learned to use their bodies to refute domestic destiny, beauty offered women new ways to envision and to assert themselves. Thus through rituals of making up and making over, French women made beauty, as a strategy and as a contradiction, central to the production, practice, and performance of femininity.

Notes

INTRODUCTION

1. Comtesse de Norville, *Les coulisses de la beauté: Comment la femme séduit* (Paris: S. Ampleman, 1895), 157.

2. Ibid.

3. Sylvie, *Comment je fais ma beauté* (Paris: Éditions de "femme de France," 1937).

4. Georges Vigarello, *Histoire de la beauté: Le Corps, et l'art d'embellir de la Renaissance à nos jours* (Paris: Éditions du seuil, 2004), 135–36, 138.

5. Jacques Pinset and Yvonne Deslandres, *Histoire des soins de beauté* (Paris: Presses universitaires de France, 1960), 93; Valerie Steele, *Fashion and Eroticism: Ideals of Feminine Beauty from the Victorian Era to the Jazz Age* (New York: Oxford University Press, 1985), 118.

6. Steele, *Fashion and Eroticism,* 218.

7. Corset estimation from Vigarello, *Histoire de la beauté,* 161.

8. Steele, *Fashion and Eroticism,* 213, 221.

9. Morag Martin, *Selling Beauty: Cosmetics, Commerce, and French Society, 1750–1830* (Baltimore: Johns Hopkins University Press, 2009), 104; Georges Vigarello, *Concepts of Cleanliness: Changing Attitudes in France since the Middle Ages,* trans. Jean Birrell (Cambridge: Cambridge University Press, 1988), 132.

10. Vigarello, *Concepts of Cleanliness,* 112–13, 114, 137.

11. Judith Butler, "Performative Acts and Gender Constitution: An Essay in Phenomenology and Feminist Theory," in *Performing Feminisms: Feminist Critical Theory and the Theatre,* ed. Sue Ellen Case (Baltimore: Johns Hopkins University Press, 1990), 282.

12. In *Émile,* Rousseau describes those "foppish manikins" who enjoy the luxuries of effeminate fashions as "a disgrace to their own sex and to the sex which they imitate" (J-J Rousseau, *Émile,* trans. Barbara Foxley [London: Dent; New York: Dutton, 1963], 328).

13. Michael Kwass, "Big Hair: A Wig History of Consumption in Eighteenth-Century France," *American Historical Review* 111, no. 3 (June 2006): 631–59.

14. James F. McMillan, *France and Women 1789–1914: Gender, Society and Politics* (London: Routledge, 2000), 10–11; Rousseau, *Émile,* 371–72.

15. Morag Martin, "Consuming Beauty," 131–32.

16. Ibid., 111. See also "The Bad Mother," in Lynn Hunt, *The Family Romance of the French Revolution* (Berkeley: University of California Press, 1992), 89–123.

17. Rousseau, *Émile,* 322, 328.

18. Ibid., 331; Morag Martin, "Consuming Beauty," 141, 142.

19. Mary Lynn Stewart, *For Health and Beauty: Physical Culture for Frenchwomen, 1880s–1930s* (Baltimore: Johns Hopkins University Press, 2000); Vigarello, *Histoire de la beauté.*

20. Butler, "Performative Acts," 274.

21. Simone de Beauvoir, *The Second Sex,* trans. H. M. Parshley (New York: Vintage, 1952), 588–618; see also Thorstein Veblen, *Theory of the Leisure Class* (London: Sage, 1970), 127.

22. Beauvoir, *The Second Sex,* 589.

23. Anne Anlin Cheng, "Wounded Beauty: An Exploratory Essay on Race, Feminism, and the Aesthetic Question," *Tulsa Studies in Women's Literature* 19, no. 2 (Autumn 2000): 191.

24. To "mend" this damage, some feminists propose a return to a "natural" body located outside of the capitalist economy (see N.C. Baker, *The Beauty Trap* [New York: Franklin Watts, 1984]; S. Brownmiller, *Femininity* [New York: Linden, 1984]; and R. Coward, *Female Desire: Women's Sexuality Today* [London: Paladin, 1984]). Llewellyn Negrin provides an insightful overview of these and other works devoted to this subject in her article "The Self as Image: A Critical Appraisal of Postmodern Theories of Fashion," *Theory, Culture & Society* 163, no. 3 (1999): 99–118. Other scholars have focused on the performance opportunities opened to women by beauty work (see K. Silverman, "Fragments of a Fashionable Discourse," in *Studies in Entertainment,* ed. T. Modleski [Bloomington: Indiana University Press, 1986], 139–54; and Elizabeth Wilson, *Adorned in Dreams: Fashion and Modernity* [London: Virago, 1987]). Some continue to regard the beauty industry as harmful to women (see Sandra Lee Bartky, *Femininity and Domination* [New York: Routledge, 1990]; and Naomi Wolf, *The Beauty Myth: How Images of Beauty Are Used Against Women* [New York: William Morrow, 1991]).

25. Laws passed in 1881 and 1886 enabled women to establish their own savings accounts without a husband's authorization or intervention; the Naquet Law of 1884 reintroduced woman's right to divorce; and in 1907, women gained the right to use their earnings as they saw fit. The See Law in 1880 established secondary schools for girls, and under the Ferry Laws of 1881 and 1882, compulsory, free education became available to all.

26. M. Featherstone, "The Body in Consumer Culture," in *The Body: Social Process and Cultural Theory,* ed. Featherstone, Mike Hepworth, and Bryan S. Turner, 170–96 (London: Sage, 1991); J. Finkelstein, *The Fashioned Self* (Oxford: Polity, 1991); Butler, "Performative Acts," 270–82.

27. Ilya Parkins, *Poiret, Dior, and Schiaparelli: Fashion, Femininity, and Modernity* (New York: Berg, 2012), 4.

28. Danielle Allérès, *Industrie cosmétique: Art-beauté-culture* (Paris: Economica, 1986).

29. Bruno Abescat, *La saga des Bettencourt, L'Oréal: Une fortune française* (Paris: Plon, 2002); Elisabeth Barillé, *Coty: Parfumeur et visionnaire* (Paris: Éditions Assouline, 1995); François Dalle, *L'aventure L'Oréal* (Paris: Odile Jacob, 2001); Marcel Haedrich, *Coco Chanel: Her Life, Her Secrets* (Boston: Little, Brown, 1972); Lee Israel, *Estée Lauder: Beyond the Magic* (New York: Macmillan, 1985); Delphine David, *La distribution de parfums et produits de beauté: Quelle redistribution des cartes?* (Paris: Institut Xerfi, Conjuncture secteurs d'entreprise & recherches financières, April 1997); Jean-Michel Hautefort, *Parfumerie-cosmétique: Les nouveaux enjeux* (Paris: Eurostaf–Les echos études, 2000); Christophe Roquilly, *Le droit des produits cosmétiques* (Paris: Economica, 1991); Louis Bergeron, *Les industries du luxe en France* (Paris: Éditions Odile Jacob, 1998); Paul Gerbod, "Les coiffeurs en France (1800–1950)," *Le mouvement social,* no. 14 (January–March 1981): 71–85; Michèle Ruffat, "La recherche historique sur l'industrie pharmaceutique en France et à l'étranger," *Revue d'hstoire de la pharmacie,* no. 305 (1995); Michèle Ruffat, *175 Years of French*

Pharmaceutical Industry: History of Synthélabo (Paris: Éditions la découverte, 1996); Steven Zdatny, *Fashion, Work, and Politics in Modern France* (New York: Palgrave Macmillan, 2006); Claudine Chevrel and Béatrice Cornet, *Grain de beauté: Un siècle de beauté par la publicité* (Paris: Somogy éditions d'art, Bibliothèque Forney, 1993); F. Ghozland and J-P Forestier, *Cosmétiques être et paraître* (Milan: Éditions Milan, 1987).

30. Kathy Peiss, *Hope in a Jar: The Making of America's Beauty Culture* (New York: Henry Holt, 1998), 6; Lois Banner, *American Beauty* (Chicago: University of Chicago Press, 1984).

31. See Victoria De Grazia, *The Sex of Things: Gender and Consumption in Historical Perspective,* with Ellen Furlough (Berkeley: University of California Press, 1996); Susan Strasser, Charles McGovern, and Matthias Judt, eds., *Getting and Spending: European and American Consumer Societies in the Twentieth Century* (New York: Cambridge University Press, 1998); and Vanessa Schwartz, *Spectacular Realities: Early Mass Culture in Fin-de-Siècle Paris* (Berkeley: University of California Press, 1998).

32. Celia Lury, *Consumer Culture* (New Brunswick, N.J.: Rutgers University Press, 1996), 1, 7, 9; Jean Baudrillard, "Consumer Society," in *Selected Writings,* 32–59 (Stanford, Calif.: Stanford University Press, 2002).

33. See, for example, Vigarello, *Histoire de la beauté.*

34. Mary Lynn Stewart explains the "new standards of cleanliness" in *For Health and Beauty.*

35. Butler, "Performative Acts," 270.

36. Kathleen Canning, *Gender History in Practice: Historical Perspectives on Bodies, Class, and Citizenship* (Ithaca, N.Y.: Cornell University Press, 2006), 28.

PART I

1. Charles Baudelaire, "In Praise of Cosmetics," in *The Painter of Modern Life and Other Essays,* trans. and ed. Jonathan Mayne (New York: Phaidon, 1964), 33, 34.

2. Stephen Gundle, *Glamour: A History* (New York: Oxford University Press, 2008), 9–10.

CHAPTER ONE

1. Dr. Paul Marrin, *La beauté chez l'homme et chez la femme: Les moyens de l'acquérir, de la conserver, de l'augmenter,* 15th ed. (Paris: Ernest Kolb, 1891), 10.

2. Karen Offen, "Depopulation, Nationalism, and Feminism in Fin-de-Siècle France," *American Historical Review* 89, no. 3 (1984): 652.

3. Arthur Marwick, *Beauty in History: Society, Politics, and Personal Appearance c. 1500 to the Present* (London: Thames and Hudson, 1985), 220.

4. Jack D. Ellis, *The Physician-Legislators of France: Medicine and Politics in the Early Third Republic, 1870–1914* (Cambridge: Cambridge University Press, 1990), 6.

5. Ibid., 2, 5.

6. Ibid., 6–12.

7. Jan Goldstein, "Foucault among the Sociologists: The "Disciplines" and the History of the Professions," *History and Theory* 23, no. 2 (May 1984): 170–92.

8. Offen, "Depopulation, Nationalism," 137.

9. Robert Nye, *Crime, Madness, and Politics in Modern France: The Medical Concept of National Decline* (Princeton, N.J.: Princeton University Press, 1984), 161, 163.

10. Examples include Arsène Dumont, *Dépopulation et civilisation: Étude démographique* (Paris: Lecrosnier et Babé, 1890); René Gonnard, *La dépopulation en France* (Lyon, 1898); René Lavollée, *Études de morale sociale: Lectures et conférences* (Paris: Guillaumin, 1897); and Edme Piot, *La question de la dépopulation en France: Le mal, ses causes, ses remèdes* (Paris: Société anonyme de publications périodiques, 1900).

11. Offen, "Depopulation, Nationalism," 651. Offen's estimate includes the 1.6 million French relocated in the German annexation of Alsace and Lorraine.

12. David Pomfret, "'A Muse for the Masses': Gender, Age, and Nation in France, Fin de Siècle," *American Historical Review* 109, no. 4 (December 2004): 1441.

13. Nye, *Crime, Madness, and Politics,* 134.

14. Alain Corbin, *Le miasme et la jonquille: L'odorat et l'imaginaire social XVIIIe–XIXe siècles* (Paris: Aubier Montaigne, 1982), 179.

15. Ghozland and Forestier, *Cosmétiques être et paraître,* 52.

16. Most rural French did not have indoor plumbing until the 1950s, and in 1900, fewer than 4 percent of Parisian homes had bathtubs; even fewer had hot-water heaters. The first nationwide disinfection campaign occurred under the July Monarchy as a response to the cholera epidemic. Scenes devoted to hygiene science and to demonstrating sanitary techniques (e.g., indoor plumbing, water filtration, vaccination, and disinfecting surfaces) occupied space at the Universal Exposition for the first time in 1900 (Ministère du commerce, de l'industrie des postes et des télégraphes, *Exposition universelle internationale de 1900: Rapports du jury international, Group XVI—Économique sociale.—Hygiène—Assistance publique* [Paris: Imprimerie nationale, 1900]).

17. Ris-Paquot, *Hygiène, médicine, parfumerie, pharmacie* (Paris: Librairie Renouard, 1894), 17.

18. Ernest Monin, *L'hygiène de la beauté: Formulaire Cosmétique* (Paris: Octave Doin, 1896), 46–47.

19. Ibid., 13.

20. César Gardeton, *Dictionnaire de la beauté: La toilette sans danger* (Paris, 1827).

21. Ris-Paquot, *Hygiène, médicine, parfumerie, pharmacie.*

22. Monin, *L'hygiène de la beauté,* 79, 105.

23. Ernest Monin, *Hygiène de la femme: Précepts médicaux pratiques pour le teint, la peau, les dents, la chevelure* (Paris: Flammarion, 1894).

24. Doctoresse M. Schultz, *Hygiène générale de la femme: Alimentation—vêtements—soins corporels d'après l'enseignement et la pratique du Docteur Auvard* (Paris: Octave Doin, 1903), 2, 312.

25. Ibid., 6–7.

26. A notable eighteenth-century exception to this is Albert Le Camus's *Abdeker* (1754).

27. Monin, *L'hygiène de la beauté,* 107, 159–60, 177, 110, 114, 29.

28. Marrin, *La beauté chez,* 184, 169, 184, 171, 183, 13.

29. Vigarello, *Histoire de la beauté,* 180. Because the category "parfumerie" increasingly included other beauty aids, it is difficult to discern if these figures strictly reflect perfume sales, or if they are intended to apply to cosmetics as well. Vigarello's source—A. Picard, *Exposition internationale de 1900, le billon d'une siècle* (Paris, 1906)—is unclear.

30. Value here reflects a current franc value rather than a constant franc value; therefore, it does not measure for franc inflation and deflation in this period. It is intended to suggest, rather, that perfumery sales significantly increased between the July Monarchy and the Second Empire

(two periods that tolerated cosmetic use) and between the Second Empire and the Third Republic to demonstrate increasing demand.

31. The state and its administrative bodies began to regulate cosmetics production in the mid-1700s. After 1765, the *Dictionnaire d'histoire naturelle* warned against metallic substances in cosmetics manufacture; after 1770, inventors were frequently called in front of L'Académie des sciences; and in 1778, the king created la Société royale de médecine to monitor *"remèdes secrets."*

32. Danielle Allérès, *Industrie cosmétique: Art-beauté-culture* (Paris: Economica, 1986), 12, 29. Zinc oxide replaced dangerous lead/copper mixtures as a preservative in facial powders. Petroleum allowed for longer product storage than traditional, organic greases. Vaseline petroleum jelly was patented in 1878.

33. Eric Fouassier, "Le cadre général de la loi du 21 Germinal An XI," March 2003, www.ordre.pharmacien.fr Documents de référence—Histoire et art pharmaceutique; Christine Debue-Barazer, "Le médicament 1803–1940," March 2003, www.ordre.pharmacien.fr, 1–5 Documents de référence—Histoire et art pharmaceutique.

34. Paul Gerbord, "Les coiffeurs en France (1800–1950)," *Le mouvement social,* no. 14 (January–March 1981): 71. Examples of journals and reviews include A. Mallemont, *Manuel de la coiffure des dames* (Paris: E. Robinet, 1898). The most prolific magazine was Eugène Schueller's *La coiffure de Paris* (1908), later *Votre beauté.*

35. Jacques Dhur, "Coiffeurs et pharmaciens," *La parfumerie moderne,* no. 1 (January 1910): 88–89.

36. Ibid., 88.

37. André Langrand, response to Jacques Dhur, *La parfumerie moderne,* no. 1 (January 1910): 89.

38. Abescat, *La saga des Bettencourt.*

39. In 1939, following a merger with a $135,000 start-up, Schueller made L'Oreal a limited liability corporation (Randall K. Morck, ed., *A History of Corporate Governance around the World: Family Business Groups and Professional Managers* [Chicago: University of Chicago Press, 2005], 210).

40. The *Wall Street Journal* listed L'Oreal as the seventy-first-largest global public company based on its $47 billion market value in August 2003. Sales for L'Oreal reached $15 billion in 2002 (Morck, *A History of Corporate Governance,* 210).

41. Lisa Tiersten, *Marianne in the Market: Envisioning Consumer Society in Fin-de-Siècle France* (Berkeley: University of California Press, 2001), 7.

42. Michael Miller, *Au Bon Marché: Bourgeois Culture and the Department Store, 1869–1920* (Princeton, N.J.: Princeton University Press, 1981), 54, 167, 181, 230, 50–52.

43. Erika Diane Rappaport, *Shopping for Pleasure: Women in the Making of London's West End* (Princeton, N.J.: Princeton University Press, 2000).

44. Rosalind H. Williams, *Dream Worlds: Mass Consumption in Late Nineteenth-Century France* (Berkeley: University of California Press, 1982).

45. Linda Clark, "Bringing Feminine Qualities in the Public Sphere: The Third Republic's Appointment of Female Inspectors," in *Gender and the Politics of Social Reform in France, 1870–1914,* ed. Elinor Acampo, 128–56 (Baltimore: Johns Hopkins University Press, 1995), 129, 146.

46. Pinset and Deslandres, *Histoire des soins,* 108.

47. Gundle, *Glamour,* 389.

48. Gerbod, "Les coiffeurs en France (1800–1950)," 72–73.

49. Ibid.

50. Piess, *Hope in a Jar,* 95.

51. Marc Martin, "Structures de societé et consciences rebelles: Les resistances à la publicité dans la France de l'entre-deux guerres," *Le mouvement social* 146 (January–March 1989): 27–40.

52. Clark Hultquist, "The Price of Dreams: A History of Advertising in France, 1927–1968" (Ph.D., Ohio State University, 1996), 2, 2–3.

53. J. Arren, *Sa majesté la publicité* (Tours: Alfred Marne, 1914), 9. On consumer psychology, see Jules Lapin, "Nos conferences: La psychologie dans les affaires," *Commerce et industrie*, no. 20 (March 20, 1909): 100–105. On periodical advertising, see C. Espinadel, "Les médiums de la publicité: Les périodiques," *Commerce et industrie* 32 (January 20, 1910): 15–17.

54. René Miquel, "Vos vitrines," *La coiffure de Paris*, 1929, 38.

55. Corbin, *The Foul and the Fragrant*, 199.

56. *Fleur de Bouquet* image reproduced from Ghozland and Forestier, *Cosmétiques être et paraître*, 87.

57. Diane Barthel, *Putting on Appearances: Gender and Advertising* (Philadelphia: Temple University Press, 1988), 39.

58. Crème Simon ad reproduced from Ghozland and Forestier, *Cosmétiques etre et paraître*, 73.

59. Lait des Alpes ad, reproduced from Ghozland and Forestier, *Cosmétiques être et paraître*, 73.

60. Autard, *Femina* 1908.

61. Nover, Je n'emploie que les produits de la parfumerie Idea, ca. 1900, in Chevrel and Cornet, *Grain de beauté*, 180.

62. Anonyme, Parfumerie Gellé frères, ca, 1893, in Chevrel and Cornet, *Grain de beauté*, 127.

63. Anonyme, Parfumerie Félix Potin, 1893, in Chevrel and Cornet, *Grain de beauté*, 125.

64. Jules Chéret, Cosmydor savon, se vend partout. Paris, impr., Chaix, 1891

65. Jules Chéret, La Diaphane: Poudre de riz, Sarah Bernhardt, in Chevrel and Cornet, *Grain de beauté*, 140.

66. Margaret Beetham, *A Magazine of Her Own? Domesticity and Desire in the Woman's Magazine, 1800–1914* (London: Routledge, 1996), 145.

CHAPTER TWO

1. André-Valdès, *Encyclopédie illustrée des élégances: Hygiène de la beauté* (Paris: Librairie Marpon et Flammarion, 1892), 104, 105.

2. My emphasis.

3. André-Valdès, *Encyclopédie illustrée des élégances*, 4.

4. Theresa Braunschneider, "The People That Things Make: Coquettes and Consumer Culture in Early Eighteenth-Century British Satire," in *Refiguring the Coquette: Essays on Culture and Coquetry*, ed. Shelley King and Yael Schlick, 39–61 (Lewisburg, Pa.: Bucknell University Press, 2008).

5. *Olympia* was completed in 1863 (the same year that *Le figaro* published Baudelaire's "Painter of Modern Life") but not shown until 1865. Carol Armstrong, *Manet Manette* (New Haven: Yale University Press, 2002); Charles Bernheimer, "Manet's *Olympia:* The Figuration of Scandal," *Poetics Today* 10, no. 2 (Summer 1989): 255–77; Charles Bernheimer, *Figures of Ill-Repute: Representing Prostitution in Nineteenth-Century France* (Durham, N.C.: Duke University Press, 1997); T. J. Clark, *The Painting of Modern Life: Paris in the Art of Manet and His Followers* (New York: Knopf, 1985); Laurie Teal, "The Hollow Women: Modernism, the Prostitute, and Commodity Aesthetics," *Differences* 3, no. 3 (Fall 1995): 80–108.

6. Cited in Bernhiemer, "Manet's Olympia," 265.

7. Viewers, according to Bernhiemer, "acted as if they were trapped by this provocative image" and responded to it "only with derisive hostility and contempt" (ibid.).

8. Clark, *The Painting of Modern Life,* 84.

9. Review cited ibid., 83.

10. Edmond de Goncourt's *La Fille Ellsa* (1877); J. K. Huysmans's *Marthe, histoire d'une fille* (1876); Pol de Saint-Merry, *Petite bibliothèque du coeur* (Paris: H. Geoffroy, 1898)—Two of the twelve volumes of this series, "Le péché" and "Pécheresses," are devoted to prostitutes; Armand Silvestre, *Le péché d'Eve* (1885); and Emile Zola's *La confession de Claude* (1865).

11. Clark, *The Painting of Modern Life,* 88.

12. Ibid., 132.

13. Ibid., 83.

14. Émile Zola, *Nana,* trans. Douglas Parmée (New York: Oxford University Press, 1992), xxvi.

15. Mary Louise Roberts, "Gender, Consumption and Commodity Culture," *American Historical Review* 103, no. 3 (June 1998): 818.

16. Émile Zola, *Nana* (Paris: G. Charpentier, et. Cie Éditeurs, 1888), 18; hereafter cited parenthetically.

17. Armstrong, *Manet,* 228.

18. Abigail Solomon Godeau, "The Other Side of Venus: The Visual Economy of Feminine Display," in *The Sex of Things: Gender and Consumption in Historical Perspective,* ed. Victoria De Grazia with Ellen Furlough (Berkeley: University of California Press, 1996), 128.

19. Emily Apter, "Cabinet Secret: Fetishism, Prostitution, and the Fin-de-Siècle Interior," *Assemblage,* no. 9 (June 1989): 9.

20. Solomon Godeau, "The Other Side of Venus."

21. Mary Lynn Stewart, *Dressing Modern Frenchwomen: Marketing, Haute Couture, 1919–1939* (Baltimore: Johns Hopkins University Press, 2008), 112.

22. Lenard R. Berlanstein, "Historicizing and Gendering Celebrity Culture: Famous Women in Nineteenth-Century France," *Journal of Women's History* 16, no. 4 (Winter 2004): 81.

23. Stewart, *Dressing the Modern French Woman,* 61.

24. "Le type idéal de la jeune fille française," *Femina,* February, 1, 1908, 54; "Le type idéal de la jeune fille française," *Femina,* February 15, 1908, 76.

25. Cécile Sorel, "Les grandes coquettes," *Femina,* February 1, 1908, 60.

26. "'No One Shall Make Fun of My Divine Beauty': Infuriated by the Caricature of Herself at the Comic Artists' Exhibition, Mlle. Cecile Sorel, the Famous French Beauty, Smashes the Horrid Picture with Her Jewelled Bon-bon Box," *Pittsburg Post Gazette,* May 29, 1921, 84.

27. Ibid.

28. Maurice Ravidat, "Chez la manicure," *Femina,* September 15, 1902.

29. Myiad, "L'art du maquillage," *Femina,* March 15, 1903, 475, 476.

30. Harriet Meta Smith ad, *Femina,* February 15, 1910, xxiii.

31. Octave Uzanne, *Fashion in Paris: The Various Phases of Feminine Taste and Aesthetics from 1797 to 1897,* trans. Lady Mary Loyd (London: Heinemann; New York: Scribner's Sons, 1898), 175.

32. This move distanced high-class courtesans and actresses from common sex workers, who were regarded as unhygienic and vulgar.

33. Leonard Berlanstein, *Daughters of Eve: A Cultural History of French Theater Women from the Old Regime to the Fin-de-Siècle* (Cambridge: Harvard University Press, 2004), 218, 110, 32.

34. Gundle, *Glamour,* 139.

35. Marwick, *Beauty in History,* 291.

36. "Le concours international de beauté," *Femina,* September 1907, 407.

37. Pomfret, "The People's Muse."

38. Elizabeth K. Menon, *Evil by Design: The Creation and Marketing of the Femme Fatale* (Urbana: University of Illinois Press, 2006), 174. In her history of the femme fatale, Menon provides a lengthy and insightful discussion of women as dolls.

39. Dolls were popular toys before this time; however, *poupées à la mode* were elaborately dresses, well-coiffed, and painted in full makeup. They were dolls intended to convey the norms of fashion and beauty (Menon, *Evil by Design,* 169–72).

40. Comtesse de Gencé, *Le cabinet de toilette d'une honnête femme* (Paris: Bibliothèque des ouvrages pratiques, 1909); Norville, *Les coulisses de la beauté;* Baronne Staffe, *Brevet de femme chic* (Paris: Flammarion, 1907); Comtesse de Tramar, *Le bréviaire de la femme: Pratiques secrets de la beauté* (Paris: Victor-Havard 1903).

41. Tramar, *Le bréviaire de la femme,* 33.

42. Gencé, *Le cabinet de toilette,* 7.

43. Staffe, *Brevet de femme chic,* 59.

44. Norville, *Les coulisses de la beauté,* 6; Tramar, *Le bréviaire de la femme,* 46.

45. Baronne Staffe, *Mes secrets pour plaire et pour très aimé* (Paris: Les éditions 1900, 1900); Norville, *Les coulisses de la beauté,* 5, 67.

46. Baronne Staffe, *Le cabinet de toilette* (Paris: Victor-Havard, 1891), 3.

47. Comtesse de Tramar, *A la conquête du bonheur!* (Paris: A. Maloine, 1912); Tramar, *Le bréviaire de la femme,* 12–13, 118.

48. Ibid., 33.

49. Staffe, *Le cabinet de toilette,* 5.

50. Vicomtesse Nacla, *Le boudoir: Conseils d'élégance* (Paris: Librairie Ernest Flammarion, 1896), 259.

51. André-Valdès, *Encyclopédie illustrée des élégances,* 56. The author recommended one bath per week in fresh water.

52. Ibid., 8.

53. Tramar, *Le bréviaire de la femme,* 38.

54. Baronne Staffe, *La femme dans la famille* (Paris: Flammarion, 1900), 3.

55. Tramar, *Que veut la femme?* 12.

56. Barthel, *Putting on Appearances,* 60.

57. Gencé, *Le cabinet de toilette,* 50.

58. Ibid., 48.

59. Nacla, *Le boudoir,* 258; Tramar, *Le bréviaire de la femme,* 61.

60. Nacla, *Le boudoir,* vi.

61. Gencé, *Le cabinet de toilette,* 7.

62. Tramar, *Le bréviaire de la femme,* 61–68.

63. Ibid., 31.

64. Gencé, *Le cabinet de toilette,* 49, 56.

65. Tramar, *A la conquête du bonheur,* 110.

66. Tramar, *Que veut la femme?* 8–9.

67. Gencé, *Le cabinet de toilette,* 56.

68. André-Valdès. *Encyclopédie illustrée des élégances,* 90–91.

69. Tramar, *Le bréviaire de la femme,* 148.

PART II

Epigraph: Colette, "Claudine Married," in *The Complete Claudine,* trans. Antonia White (New York: Farrar, Straus and Giroux, 1976), 428–29.

1. The complete Claudine series includes: *Claudine at School* (1900), *Claudine in Paris* (1901), *Claudine Married* (1902), and *Claudine and Annie* (1903).

2. Judith Thurman, *Secrets of the Flesh: A Life of Colette* (New York: Knopf, 1999).

3. Mary Louise Roberts, *Disruptive Acts: The New Woman in Fin-de-Siècle France* (Chicago: University of Chicago Press, 2002), 3–4.

4. Ibid., 7.

5. Ibid., 6.

6. For exceptions, see Roberts, *Disruptive Acts.*

7. Ibid., 3.

CHAPTER THREE

1. Colette, *Mes apprentissages,* trans. Helen Beauclerk (New York: Farrar, Straus and Giroux, 1957), 8.

2. Laurel Cummins, *Colette and the Conquest of Self* (Birmingham, Ala.: Summa, 2005); Anne Freadman, "Laurel Cummins, *Colette and the Conquest of Self,*" *French Studies* 61, no. 1 (2007): 118–19.

3. Colette, *La naissance du jour* (Paris: Flammarion, 1928); Colette, *Break of Day,* trans. Enid McLeod (New York: Farrar, Straus and Giroux, 1979), 16.

4. Colette, *Break of Day,* 35.

5. Recent examples of these works include Victoria Best, *Critical Subjectivities: Identity and Narrative in the Work of Colette and Marguerite Duras* (Bern: Peter Lang, 2000); Cummins, *Colette and the Conquest of Self;* Jerry Aline Flieger, *Colette and the Fantom Subject of Autobiography* (Ithaca, N.Y.: Cornell University Press, 1992); Claude Francis and Fernande Gontier, *Creating Colette,* vol. 2, *From Baroness to Woman of Letters, 1912–1954* (South Royalton, Vt.: Steerforth, 1999); Thurman, *Secrets of the Flesh;* and Patricia Tilburg, "Earning Her Bread: Métier, Order, and Female Honor in Colette's Music Hall, 1906–1913," *French Historical Studies* 28, no. 3 (Summer 2005): 497–530.

6.Tilburg, "Earning Her Bread."

7. Colette, *"Chéri" and "The Last of Chéri,"* trans. Richard Senhouse (New York: Penguin, 1977), 13; hereafter cited parenthetically.

8. In addition to Chéri, there are only two male characters in the novel, Léa's butler and Chéri's friend Desmond, who both play only minor roles.

9. Martina Stemberger, "*Selling Gender:* An Alternative View of 'Prostitution' in Three French Novels of the Entre-Deux-Guerres," *Neophilologus* 92 (2008): 603.

10. Ibid., 614.

11. Ibid.

12. Ibid.

13. Best, *Critical Subjectivities,* 189.

14. Ibid.

15. In 1911–12, Colette wrote four stories about Clouk and four about Chéri for *Le matin.* In the final version, Chéri has physical beauty, but he retains Clouk's self-destructiveness (Francis and Gontier, *Creating Colette,* 2:43–45).

16. Ibid., 2:6, 4.

17. Ibid., 2:6.

18. Colette quoted in *The Collected Stories of Colette,* ed. Robert Phelps, trans. Matthew Ward (New York: Farrar, Straus and Giroux, 1983).

19. On aesthetic veiling, see Flieger, *Colette and the Fantom Subject of Autobiography,* 135.

20. Best, *Critical Subjectivities,* 9.

21. Colette, *La vagabonde* (Paris: Librairie Paul Ollendorff, 1910), 4; hereafter cited parenthetically.

22. Sigmund Freud, "Three Essays on the Theory of Sexuality," in *Three Essays on the Theory of Sexuality* (1905), trans. James Strachey (New York: Basic, 2000).

23. For a more complete discussion of narcissism in a psychoanalytic frame, see Best, *Critical Subjectivities,* 190–93.

24. Irène Julièr, "Le maquillage, pratiques, discours, et interprétations" (Ph.D. diss., Paris VII, 1989), 117.

25. Colette, *The Shackle,* trans. Antonia White (New York: Farrar, Straus and Giroux, 1964), 11; hereafter cited parenthetically.

26. Melanie E. Collado, *Colette, Lucie Delarue-Mardrus, Marcelle Tinayre: Émancipation et résignation* (Paris: Harmattan, 2003), 163.

27. Colette, *Tendrils of the Vine,* quoted in Thurman, *Secrets of the Flesh,* 188

CHAPTER FOUR

Epigraph: Colette, "Le Passé," in *Paysages et portraits* (Paris: Flammarion, 1958), 11–12.

1. Tilburg, "Earning her Bread"; Tilburg, *Colette's Republic: Work, Gender, and Popular Culture in France, 1870–1914* (New York: Berghahn, 2009).

2. Roberts, *Disruptive Acts,* 11.

3. Ibid., 21.

4. Ibid., 7.

5. Colette, "Letter to Hélène Picard," in *Letters from Colette* (New York: Farrar, Straus Giroux, 1980), 96.

6. Tilburg, "Earning Her Bread."

7. Between 1907 and 1911, for example, she and Wague performed *La chair* more than three hundred times.

8. Colette, "Lettre à Georges Wague (29 avril 1909)," in *Lettres de la vagabonde,* 34.

9. Colette, *Belles Saisons: A Colette Scrapbook,* comp. Robert Phelps, trans. Matthew Ward (New York: Farrar, Straus and Giroux, 1978), 167, 175.

10. Thurman, *Secrets of the Flesh,* 303. Colette encouraged these misidentifications (Francis and Gontier, *Creating Colette,* 2:12).

11. Colette, "The Halt," in *The Collected Stories of Colette,* ed. Phelps, 105–6; hereafter cited parenthetically.

12. "The Workroom," in *The Collected Stories of Colette,* ed. Phelps, 116; hereafter cited parenthetically.

13. Colette, "Matinee," in *The Collected Stories of Colette,* ed. Phelps, 121; hereafter cited parenthetically.

14. Colette, "Love," in *The Collected Stories of Colette,* ed. Phelps, 126; hereafter cited parenthetically.

15. Cited in and Gontier, *Creating Colette,* 2:10.

16. Tilburg, *Colette's Republic,* 101.

17. Tilburg, "Earning Her Bread," 507.

18. Anne Freadman, "Breasts Are Back! Colette's Critique of Flapper Fashion," *French Studies* 60, no. 3 (2006): 346.

19. Gérard Bonal and Frédéric Maget, eds., *Colette journaliste: Chroniques et reportages 1893–1955* (Paris: Éditions du seuil, 2010), 29.

20. Despite her prolific publishing record, scant scholarly attention has been paid to Colette's journalistic works. Exceptions include Freadman, "Breasts Are Back!"; Diana Holmes, *Colette* (London: Macmillan, 1991); David Walker, *Outrage and Insight: Modern French Writers and the Fait Divers* (Oxford: Berg, 1995); and, most recently, Bonal and Maget, eds., *Colette journaliste.*

21. Thurman, *Secrets of the Flesh,* 219.

22. Colette, "Music-halls l'exilée," *Le matin,* January 27, 1911, 4.

23. Colette, "Fards," in *Demain,* June 1, 1924; republished as "Make-up," in *Journey for Myself: Selfish Memories,* trans. David Le Vey (Indianapolis: Bobbs-Merrill 1972), 70; hereafter cited parenthetically.

24. Berry points out that *Femina* could rival the most luxurious of the special edition spreads done by competitors like the *Gazette du bon ton* (1912–1925) (Berry, "Designing the Reader's Interior," 66).

25. Leonard Berlanstein, "Selling Modern Femininity: *Femina,* a Forgotten Feminist Publishing Success in Belle Époque France," *French Historical Studies* 30, no. 4 (Fall 2007): 625.

26. Ibid., 640.

27. Ibid., 628–30, 632.

28. Ibid., 640.

29. "Le livre de madame," *Femina,* June 1920.

30. Berlanstein, "Selling Modern Femininity," 627.

31. Claire Launay, "Pour qui une femme s'habille t'elle?" *Femina,* March 1920.

32. Colette, "Fards, poudres, parfums," *Femina,* November 1927, 23–25.

33. Colette, *À lettres a Hélène Picard,* 150–52.

34. In a relatively lengthy article from its March 1, 1924, issue, for example, *Vogue* told women how to be elegant with economy ("Pour être élégante avec économie," *Vogue,* March 1, 1924, 38, 50).

35. "Charm and Grace," *Vogue,* November 1, 1920; "Men's Attitudes about Women's Fashions," *Vogue,* October 1, 1920.

36. "Fards pour le soir," *Vogue,* July 1, 1929, 92; "Beauty Products," *Vogue,* September 1929.

37. Stewart, *Dressing Modern Frenchwomen,* 57.

38. I compiled the data for this table through a content analysis of each magazine, available in hard copy at the Bibliothèque Nationale de France. Any errors in counting are my own.

39. "La philosophie de la poudre et du fard," *Vogue,* March 1, 1921, 22.

40. Ibid.

41. Ibid.

42. "De l'importance d'être belle," *Vogue,* January 1, 1926, 38.

43. Ibid., 39.

44. Mme. M. T. Sylviac, "Quelques secrets sur l'art d'être belle," *Vogue,* February 1, 1924, 28–29.

45. Julier, "Le maquillage, pratiques," 99.

46. Colette, "Tomorrow's Springtime," in *Journey for Myself,* trans. Le Vey, 34; hereafter cited parenthetically.

47. Colette, "Models," in *Journey for Myself,* trans. Le Vey, 39; hereafter cited parenthetically.

48. Colette, "Elegance, Economy," cited in *Journey for Myself,* trans. Le Vey, 42; hereafter cited parenthetically.

49. Colette, *Avatars,* quoted in Thurman, *Secrets of the Flesh,* 396.

50. Julier, "Le maquillage, pratiques," 92.

51. "Le role social des instituts de beauté," *Beauté,* April 1929, 8.

52. Ibid.

53. Louis Léon-Martin, *L'industrie de la beauté* (Paris: Éditions des Portiques, 1930), 71.

54. Paul Fryer and Olga Usova, *Lina Cavalieri: The Life of Opera's Greatest Beauty, 1874–1944* (Jefferson, N.C.: McFarland, 2004), 42.

55. Ads for Cavalieri Institute, *Vogue,* 1926 (multiple issues).

56. Lina Cavalieri, *My Secrets of Beauty* (New York: Circulation Syndicate, 1914), 9.

57. Ibid., 78.

58. Piess, *Hope in a Jar,* 66.

59. Ibid., 88.

60. Lindy Woodhead, *War Paint: Madame Helena Rubinstein and Miss Elizabeth Arden: Their Lives, Their Times, Their Rivalry* (Hoboken, N.J.: Wiley, 2003), 81–82.

61. Ibid., 126.

62. Ibid.

63. Piess, *Hope in a Jar,* 89.

64. Cover reprinted in Colette, *Belles Saisons,* comp. Phelps, 102.

65. She cautioned Willy Gauither-Villars's mistress, the Chat Noir performer Charlotte Kinceler, that "glycerin ruins the hands" and recommended that she "use lanoline instead."

66. Francis and Gontier, *Creating Colette,* 2:146.

67. Ibid., 2:150.

68. Colette, *Lettres à Helene Picard,* 151.

69. Thurman, *Secrets of the Flesh,* 395.

70. Juliette Goublet, "Colette et la beauté," *Beauté-coiffure-mode* (*Votre beauté*), June 1932, 11.

71. Ibid.

72. Ibid.

73. Ibid.

74. Goudeket, *Close to Colette,* 6.

PART III

1. Dr. Nadia Grégoire Payot, *Être belle* (Paris: Presses universitaires de France, 1933).

2. Mary Louise Roberts, *Civilization without Sexes: The Great War, Cultural Crisis and the Debate on Women, 1917–1927* (Chicago: University of Chicago Press, 1994), 25–26; Françoise Thébaud, "The Great War and the Triumph of Sexual Division," in *A History of Women in the West,* 5:21–75. Women's wartime activities influenced some of their postwar civil liberties. Women could join labor unions without a husband's consent (1920), and they were permitted to take the male version of the *baccalauréat* exam (1924) (Anne-Marie Sohn, "Between the Wars in France and England," in *A History of Women in the West,* 5:114). However, French women remained disenfranchised and enjoyed limited reproductive rights (further curtailed by anti-abortion and anticontraceptive legislation passed in the early 1920s), and spouses remained legally subject to paternal authority until 1938.

3. Mary Louise Roberts, "Samson and Delilah Revisited: The Politics of Women's Fashion in 1920s France," *American Historical Review* 98, no. 3 (June 1993): 657–84; Roberts, *Civilization without Sexes,* 1994.

4. Ibid.

5. Modern Girl Around the World Research Group, "The Modern Girl Around the World: A Research Agenda and Preliminary Findings," *Gender and History* 17, no. 3 (August 2005); Modern Girl Around the World Research Group, *The Modern Girl Around the World: Consumption, Modernity, and Globalization,* ed. Alys Eve Weinbaum et al. (Durham, N.C. Duke University Press, 2008).

6. Modern Girl Around the World Research Group, *The Modern Girl Around the World,* 19.

7. Ibid., 1; Modern Girl around the World Research Group, "The Modern Girl Around the World," 245.

8. Modern Girl Around the World Research Group, *The Modern Girl Around the World,* 15.

9. Whitney Chadwick and Tirza True Latimer, eds., *The Modern Woman Revisited: Paris between the Wars* (New Brunswick, N.J.: Rutgers University Press, 2003); Roberts, *Civilization without Sexes.*

10. Modern Girl Around the World Research Group, *The Modern Girl Around the World,* 9.

CHAPTER FIVE

Parts of chapter 5 were originally as published as "Between Venus and Mercury: The 1920s Beauty Contest in France and America," *French Politics, Culture and Society* 31, no. 1 (Spring 2013): 47–68.

Epigraph: "Tires of Reigning as Queen of Beauty; Agnès Souret, Hailed as the Fairest in France, Decides to Quit Paris," *New York Times,* November 25, 1921, 18.

1. On Maria Teresa de Landa (Miss Mexico), see Victor M. Macías-González, "The Case of the Murdering Beauty: Narrative Construction, Beauty Pageants, and the Postrevolutionary Mexican National Myth, 1921–1931," in *True Stories of Crime in Modern Mexico,* ed. Robert Buffington and Pablo Piccato, 215–47 (Albuquerque: University of New Mexico Press, 2009).

2. "Paris Quarrels over Milady Beautiful," *Washington Post,* July 8, 1928, 1.

3. Chadwick and Latimer, *The Modern Woman Revisited;* Roberts, *Civilization without Sexes.*

4. Sarah Banet-Weiser, *The Most Beautiful Girl in the World: Beauty Pageants and National Identity* (Berkeley: University of California Press, 1999), 6–8; Stephen Gundle, "Feminine Beauty, National Identity, and Political Conflict in Postwar Italy, 1945–1954," *Contemporary European History* 8, no. 3 (November 1999): 378; Angela J. Latham, "Packaging Woman: The Concurrent Rise of Beauty Pageants, Public Bathing, and Other Performances of Female 'Nudity,'" *Journal of Popular Culture* 29, no. 3 (Winter 1995): 149–67; Katarina Mattsson and Katrarina Pettersson, "Crowning Miss Sweden—Constructions of Gender, Race and Nation in Beauty Pageants," paper presented at "Gender and Power in the New Europe, the Fifth European Feminist Research Conference," August 20–24, 2003, Lund University, Sweden; David Pomfret, "'A Muse for the Masses': Gender, Age, and Nation in France, Fin de Siècle," *American Historical Review* 109, no. 4 (December 2004): 1439–40; Colleen Ballerino Cohen, Richard Wilk, and Beverly Stoeltje, eds., *Beauty Queens on the Global Stage: Gender, Contests, and Power* (London: Routledge, 1996), 8–9.

5. Ballerino Cohen, Wilk, and Stoeltje, eds., *Beauty Queens on the Global Stage,* 9.

6. Banet-Weiser, *The Most Beautiful Girl in the World,* 8; Gundle, "Feminine Beauty," 378; Mattsson and Pettersson, "Crowning Miss Sweden—Constructions of Gender, Race and Nation in Beauty Pageants," 13.

7. In 1905, the *Journal* featured a series of articles authored by Emma E. Walker entitled "Pretty Girl Papers" that illustrated beauty techniques.

8. Francesca Berry, "Designing the Reader's Interior: Subjectivity and the Woman's Magazine in Early Twentieth-Century France," *Journal of Design History* 18, no. 1 (2005): 63.

9. Ibid., 74, 64; Berlanstein, "Selling Modern Femininity," 626.

10. Douglas B. Ward, "Geography of *The Ladies' Home Journal:* An Analysis of a Magazine's Audience, 1911–1955," *Journalism History* 34, no. 1 (Spring 2008): 1. The ratio of advertisements to reading material was one column to three at this time (Helen Damon-Moore, *Magazines for the Millions: Gender and Commerce in the "Ladies' Home Journal" and the Saturday Evening Post, 1880–1910* (Albany: Albany State University Press, 1994), 82, 99.

11. Bok quoted in Damon-Moore, *Magazines for the Millions,* 82.

12. Norberto Angeletti and Alberto Oliva, *In Vogue: The Illustrated History of the World's Most Famous Fashion Magazine* (New York: Rizzoli, 2006), 2, 15. See "Paris Forecast," *Vogue,* February 15, 1925.

13. Stewart, *Dressing Modern Frenchwomen,* 60.

14. Helen Chenut, *The Fabric of Gender: Working-Class Culture in Third Republic France* (State College: Pennsylvania State University Press, 2006), 308, 218n23.

15. Bread and shirt estimates from Chenut, *The Fabric of Gender,* 308; rice powder estimates from 1927 Briau agenda, commercial catalogues collection at the Bibliothèque Forney.

16. Ward, "Geography of *The Ladies' Home Journal,*" 4.

17. Banner, *American Beauty,* 381, 382.

18. "Le concours international de beauté," *Femina,* September 1907, 407.

19. Randi Hopkins, "A New Type of Queen: The Emergence of Beauty Pageants in America, 1880–1921," *Aegis* (2008): 13–15.

20. "Le concours de la plus jolie silhouette," *Vogue,* June 1, 1924, 31; "Qui a la plus jolie silhouette," *Vogue,* June 1, 1924, xxxvi; "Le concours de la que nous avons dote," *Vogue,* December 1, 1924, 26–27.

21. "Bichara l'âme du concours des plus beaux yeux de Paris les mieux maquillés," *Femina,* 1929 (multiple issues); "Concours de la Petite Reine," *Femina,* 1931 (multiple issues).

22. Peiss, *Hope in a Jar,* 215, 136. At a time when African American women were excluded from mainstream contests, the white-owned Golden Brown Company used the beauty competition to attract customers. In Italy, the toothpaste company GVM cosponsored a photo contest with the weekly *Tempo* and the women's magazine *Grazia* (Gundle, "Feminine Beauty," 367).

23. "Toute la technique du métier les concours," *La coiffure de Paris* 259 (September 1, 1931): 27–28.

24. Siân Reynolds, *France between the Wars: Gender and Politics* (London: Routledge, 1996); Roberts, *Civilization without Sexes;* Anne-Marie Sohn, "La garçonne face à l'opinion publique: Type littéraire ou type social des années 20?" *Le mouvement social* 80 (July–September 1972): 3–27; Thébaud, "Between the Wars in France and England"; Birgitte Soland, *Becoming Modern: Young Women and the Reconstruction of Womanhood in the 1920s* (Princeton, N.J.: Princeton University Press, 2000).

25. Despite the growing acceptance and popularity of beauty contests, some groups vociferously opposed them. In 1922, an American woman's league accused the Miss America Pageant of insulting womanhood and endangering the nation's morals (Ballerino Cohen, Wilk, and Stoeltje, eds., *Beauty Queens on the Global Stage,* 7).

26. On Bastille Day festivities, see Charles Rearick, "Festivals in Modern France: The Experience of the Third Republic," *Journal of Contemporary History* 12 (1977): 435–60; and Rosemonde Sanson, *Le 14 Juillet: Fête et conscience nationale, 1789–1965* (Paris: Flammarion, 1976).

27. Pomfret, "A Muse for the Masses," 1443, 1444.

28. Ibid., 1445.

29. Banner, *American Beauty,* chap. 12; Hopkins, "A New Type of Queen"; *American Experience: Miss America,* PBS, www.pbs.org/wgbh/amex/missamerica.

30. Latham, "Packaging Woman," 163.

31. Maurice de Waleffe, *Quand Paris était un paradis, mémoires, 1900–1939* (Paris: Société des éditions Denoël, 1947), 445.

32. This figure has also been quoted by de Waleffe himself as 190,000 votes. I have chosen to go with the more modest number, given de Waleffe's proclivity for exaggeration.

33. Ibid., 445–46. Sadly, Souret died in Argentina in 1928 of peritonitis at age twenty-six.

34. "Tires of Reigning as Queen of Beauty," 18.

35. Aro Velmet, "Beauty and Big Business: Gender, Race, and Civilizational Decline at French Beauty Pageants, 1920–1938," *French History* 28 (1), March 2014, 66–91.

36. Bill Cherry, "Miss America Was Once Pageant of Pulchritude," *Galveston Daily News,* October 25, 2004.

37. The other countries invited to participate were Cuba, Italy, Luxembourg, Portugal, and Spain.

38. De Waleffe, *Quand Paris était un paradis,* 447.

39. Maurice de Waleffe, "Miss France en Amérique," *Le journal,* Fonds Rondel, Bibliothèque Arsenal.

40. "Thousands Greet First Pageant Arrivals When Cuba Brings Eight Entries," *Galveston Daily News,* June 1, 1928, 1.

41. "Estimate of Revue Crowd Is 150,000," *Galveston Daily News,* June 4, 1928, 2.

42. Stanley E. Babb, "Jupe Pluvis Redeems Self for Saturday Washout with Perfect Weather for Parade," *Galveston Daily News,* June 4, 1928, 2; Revue Entries Are Loudly Acclaimed in Opening Parade," *Galveston Daily News,* June 4, 1928, 2.

43. "They Picked Miss Universe," *Galveston Daily News,* June 6, 1928, 2; "National Traits Asserted in Reaction of Beauties to Victories in Pageant," *Galveston Daily News,* June 6, 1928, 2.

44. "National Traits Asserted in Reaction of Beauties to Victories in Pageant," *Galveston Daily News,* June 6, 1928, 1.

45. "Paris Quarrels over Milady Beautiful," *Washington Post,* July 8, 1928.

46. Ibid. Jenny operated her fashion house in Paris from 1908 to 1938.

47. Ibid.

48. "Miss United States Expresses Surprise at Winning Award," *Galveston Daily News,* June 5, 1928, 1.

49. "Paris Quarrels over Milady Beautiful."

50. Because of World War II, France did not host a pageant from 1941 to 1946, and, for financial reasons, the Miss Universe Pageant was discontinued between 1935 and 1952.

51. Jackie Stacey, *Star Gazing: Hollywood Cinema and Female Spectatorship* (London: Routledge, 1994), 180.

52. Juliette Goublet, "Madame Cécile Sorel parle de la beauté," *Beauté-coiffure-mode,* April 1, 1932, 9.

53. Liane de Pougy, *My Blue Notebooks: The Intimate Journal of Paris's Most Beautiful and Notorious Courtesan* (New York: Tarcher/Putnam Press, 1979), 49.

54. Caroline Otero, *My Story* (London: A. M. Philpot, 1927), 204.

55. "Elles seraient plus jolies si . . . ," *Votre beauté,* May 1936, 52–53, 63.

56. "Le conseils de Mlle. Fanny Ward," *Femina,* January 1929, 16–19.

57. Gisèle de Birzville, "Le maquillage en 10 minutes," *Pour vous,* October 19, 1934.

58. Vigarello, *Histoire de beauté,* 207–8.

59. "Si vous changez votre type . . . les vedettes le font bien," *Votre beauté,* November 1938, 18–21.

60. "Secrets de stars," *Vogue,* September 1, 1936.

61. Stacey, *Star Gazing,* 180.

62. Richard Kuisel, *Seducing the French: The Dilemma of Americanization* (Berkeley: University of California Press, 1997), 10–11.

63. Brooks's wardrobe was designed by French designer Jean Patou.

64. Sarah Berry, *Screen Style: Fashion and Femininity in 1930s Hollywood.* (Minneapolis: University of Minnesota Press, 2000), 61, 82.

65. This resembled real pageants. As Stanley Babb commented during the 1928 Miss Universe Pageant: "The crowd presented a gorgeously colored spectacle of humanity. It was orderly—surprisingly so—it was thoroughly good natured." Nonetheless, there were some "wisecrackers" in attendance who "found an appreciative and uncritical audience for their sallies and comments" (Stanley E. Babb, "Jupe Pluvis Redeems Self for Saturday Washout with Perfect Weather for Parade," *Galveston Daily News,* June 4, 1928, 2).

66. "Pageant Beauties Leaving for Home; Miss Italy Is Given Favorable Contract," *Galveston Daily News,* June 8, 1928, 1.

67. Tracy Cox points out that this song recalls Brooks's first role as a beauty contestant in *The*

American Venus (1926) (Tracy Cox, "Consuming Distractions in *Prix de beauté*," *Camera Obscura* 50 17, no. 2 [2002]: 47).

68. Susan Dworkin, *Miss America, 1945: Bess Myerson's Own Story* (New York: New Market Press, 1988), 64.

69. Pomfret, "The Peoples' Muse," 1462.

70. Mary Ann Doane, *Femmes Fatales: Feminism, Film Theory, Psychoanalysis.* (London: Routledge, 1991), 77; Cox, "Consuming Distractions in *Prix de beauté*," 45–46.

71. Claude Doré, "Du film ironique au film dramatique: Les projets de René Clair," *Ciné-Miroir,* June 7, 1929.

72. Ibid., 58. Brooks was also cast as Lulu in George Pabst's German production *Pandora's Box* (1928).

CHAPTER SIX

Epigraph: Phyllis Earle, "Ce que doit être le maquillage moderne," *Vogue,* December 1, 1927.

1. Ibid.

2. Mary Nolan, *Visions of Modernity: American Business and the Modernization of Germany* (New York: Oxford University Press, 1994); Strasser, McGovern, and Judt, eds., *Getting and Spending.* On advertisers, see Marjorie Beale, *The Modernist Enterprise: French Elites and the Threat of Modernity, 1900–1940* (Stanford, Calif.: Stanford University Press, 1999).

3. Modern Girl Around the World Research Group, "The Modern Girl Around the World," 287.

4. Created by the New York pharmacist Theron T. Pond in 1846, Pond's cold creams and vanishing creams were available in France by 1914. French consumers could purchase Pepsodent by 1918, although the company marketed exclusively to wealthy consumers during this period. In the 1920s, the Colgate Company, which sold Palmolive soap, began establishing operations throughout Europe.

5. Dorothy Gray, the salon first established in New York City in 1916, occupied 34 avenue George V; Revlon was at 42 rue de la Boétie; Ayer was located at 33 boulevard Haussmann; and Earle at 15 rue de la Paix.

6. www.Coty.com.

7. *Vogue,* October 1, 1930, 5.

8. L'Oréal published several one-page ad/articles like the one entitled "L'Oréal defend la teinture pour cheveux. Un procès ridicule.—Attitude hostile et intellegente de la presse—La réponse de L'Oréal" in *La coiffure de Paris* throughout the period, attempting to allay the safety concerns of both its professional clients and its product consumers (*La coiffure de Paris* 228 [February 1, 1929]). See also "Les décolorations rapides l'oréal blanc," *La coiffure de Paris* 267 (May 15, 1932), in which the company responds to purchaser letters. "Une grande entreprise Française," *La coiffure de Paris: Revue professionnelle illustrée. artistique, littéraire, scientifique* 238 (December 1929), 24.

9. Abescat, *La saga des Bettencourt.*

10. *Votre beauté* grew out of Schueller's trade journal *Coiffure de Paris* (1909).

11. Danielle Allérès, *Industrie cosmetique: Art-beauté-culture* (Paris: Economica, 1986), 61–62.

12. Crème Activa ad, *Femina,* July 1922.

13. Kemolite ad, *Vogue,* December 1, 1927.

14. Odorono ad, *Vogue,* 1926 (multiple issues).

15. Odorono and Pepsodent are available today for purchase in drugstores.

16. Le Dentol ad, *Femina,* September 1922; Pepsodent, *Femina,* 1929 (multiple issues); and Bi-Oxyne, *Femina,* 1929. Many oral hygiene advertisements within women's magazines featured children, thereby reinforcing the contemporary belief that it was woman's responsibility to care for the health and hygiene of her entire family.

17. This was a relatively common practice at the time. The English firm Clark's, for example, advertised its Dyvoire system as based on "twenty-five years of investigation and discovery," and it emphasized the "scientifically-tested" quality of the kit's components (lotion, *crème rose,* and *crème grasse*).

18. Vivaudou was a popular French/American firm that featured advertisements for its creams in *Vogue, Femina,* and *Votre beauté* throughout the interwar period.

19. Vivaudou advertisement, *Vogue,* 1924 (multiple issues).

20. Ibid.

21. "Deux à trois cent millions de francs d'affaires nouvelles partager entre quelques milliers de coiffeurs: Les plus commerçants les plus actifs les plus 'à la page,'" *La coiffure de France* 268 (June 1932): 37. The article does not distinguish new and repeat users; therefore, the actual number of customers using L'Oréal hair coloring products is unclear.

22. L'Oréal ad, *Femina,* May 1922.

23. Ibid.

24. L'Oréal ad in Chevrel and Cornet, *Grain de beauté,* 39.

25. Wendy Parkins, "Moving Dangerously: Mobility and the Modern Woman," *Tulsa Studies in Women's Literature* 20, no. 1 (Spring 2001): 82.

26. Piess, *Hope in a Jar,* 103.

27. le Caméléon ad, *Vogue,* 1927 (multiple issues).

28. Delbourg-Delphis, *Le chic et le look,* 115; Crème Simon ad, *Vogue,* December 1, 1927; Crème Simon ad, *Vogue,* 1924 (multiple issues).

29. Delbourg-Delphis, *Le chic et le look,* 115.

30. Lubin advertisment, *Vogue,* 1926 (multiple issues). Pierre François Lubin founded Parfum Lubin in 1798. The perfumes were popular among elites throughout Europe (Josephine and Pauline Bonaparte wore them) and exported to America by 1830. Lubin remained a major high-end perfumer until the 1980s, when the company began manufacturing less expensive products (Edwin Morris, *Scents of Time: Perfume from Ancient Egypt to the 21st Century* [New York: Bulfinch Press, 1999]).

31. Sauzé ad, *Vogue,* 1929 (multiple issues).

32. Ibid.

33. Beale, *The Modernist Enterprise,* 47.

34. Kenneth Silver has argued that Purists, specifically Ozenfant and Le Courbusier, who authored the Purist manifesto, *La peinture moderne* (1925), sought an absolute identification between the French man and the French object (Kenneth E. Silver, "Purism: Straightening Up after the Great War," in *Modern Art and Society: An Anthology of Social and Multicultural Readings,* ed. Maurice Berger [New York: Icon Editions, 1994], 111).

35. Purists and art deco artists celebrated the durability and the stark immutability of the object. For these designers, it was not the viewer's engagement with the object, but the object itself—

the materials that composed it, the colors and lines that defined it, and the intended function of it—that made the object a thing of beauty (Silver, "Purism: Straightening Up after the Great War," 99).

36. Other compacts, for example, le Captive and Vanity Kid, were also sold in cases that were intentionally designed to double as jewelry (Delbourg-Delphis, *Le chic et le look,* 115).

37. Sauzé ad, *Vogue,* 1929 (multiple issues).

38. In 1932, the company sponsored a 20,000-franc contest in *La coiffure de Paris* asking contestants to design a *vitrine* that projected the firm's modern conception of its product (Kadeko ad, *La coiffure de Paris* 268 [May 15, 1932]: 26).

39. "L'art et la beauté rendent homage au Savon Cadum," *Vogue,* September 1, 1924.

40. Ibid.

41. Victoria de Grazia, "Changing Consumption Regimes in Europe, 1930–1970: Comparative Perspectives on the Distribution Problem," in *Getting and Spending,* ed. Strasser, McGovern, and Judt, 60–61.

42. Paul Greenhalgh, *Ephemeral Vistas: The Expositions Universelles, Great Exhibitions, and World's Fairs, 1851–1939* (New York: Manchester University Press, 1988), 3.

43. Ellen Furlough, *Consumer Cooperation in France: The Politics of Consumption, 1834–1930* (Ithaca, N.Y.: Cornell University Press, 1991), 265.

44. *La coiffure de Paris* 261 (November 1, 1931): 34.

45. It is unclear from the primary-source material exactly what purpose the *salles de fêtes* served during the show.

46. Pinset and Deslandres, *Histoire des soins de beauté,* 109.

47. Although there is no proof that Rubinstein products were tested by "dermatologists throughout the world," Rubinstein diligently tested her products. She studied dermatology in the early 1900s, and her labs supported dozens of chemists and researchers who developed hundreds of beauty products, among them the first medicated skin-care treatments.

48. Rubinstein Institute ad, *Vogue,* 1922 (multiple issues).

49. Arden Institute ad, *Vogue,* 1924 (multiple issues).

50. Phebel ad, *Vogue,* 1922 (multiple issues). Phebel, founded in Paris at the beginning of the twentieth century by Madame Marceline Sébalth, is still in operation today (see www.phebel.net/english.htm).

51. Helena Rubinstein ad, *Vogue,* 1922 (multiple issues).

52. Ibid.

53. Terminology taken from a Keva Institute Diploma from 1932, supplied to the author by Michael Semler.

54. Keva Institute, *Femina,* 1929 (multiple issues).

55. Ibid.

56. Reconstructive surgeries had been practiced for centuries, but modern plastic surgery emerged only after the Great War. The war itself proved a chief motor in the advancement of cosmetic procedures. Trench warfare left many soldiers disfigured or dismembered, and special hospitals were established in France, England, and Germany to repair deformities. These hospitals became training grounds for physicians and contributed to the emergence of cosmetic surgery as a full-fledged profession in France in the 1920s. Additionally, new anesthetic techniques and the adoption of antiseptic surgical practices (another invention of the war) made invasive procedures safer.

57. Carolyn Comisky, "Cosmetic Surgery in Paris in 1926: The Case of the Amputated Leg," *Journal of Women's History* 16, no. 3 (Fall 2004): 32. By 1930, Léon-Martin claimed that cosmetic sur-

gery was entering French morés and becoming socially accepted (Léon-Martin, *L'industrie de la beauté,* 174).

58. Dr. Suzanne Noël, *La chirurgie esthétique: Son rôle social* (Paris: Masson, 1926), cited in Comisky, "Cosmetic Surgery in Paris," 42. Noël, née Suzanne Blanche Marguerite Gros, in Laon, France, studied dermatology in 1878 and was the first female to practice cosmetic surgery in France.

59. Ibid., 45.

60. "Hygiène et beauté: 'Les instituts de beauté doivent être surveillés' déclare le Conseil supérieur d'hygiène," June 6, 1926, Dossier Beauté, Bibliothèque Marguerite Durand.

61. Ellen Furlough, "Selling the American Way in Interwar France: *Prix Uniques* and the *Salons des Arts Menagers* in Interwar France," *Journal of Social History* 26, no. 3 (Spring 1993): 496.

62. Furlough, *Consumer Cooperation in France,* 266.

63. Furlough, "Selling the American Way," 502.

64. Ibid., 498; Furlough, *Consumer Cooperation in France,* 268.

65. Furlough, "Selling the American Way in Interwar France," 496.

66. Furlough, *Consumer Cooperation in France,* 266.

67. William Leach, "Strategists of Display and the Production of Desire," in *Consuming Visions: Accumulation and Display of Goods in America, 1880–1920,* ed. Simon J. Bronner (New York: Norton, 1989), 115. As the historian Marjorie Beale has shown, despite the prewar efforts of a group of maverick advertisers affiliated with the trade journals *La publicité, Mon bureau, Atlas,* and *La publicité moderne,* "advertising posed a cultural dilemma for the French who hoped to prevent American-style commercialism from contaminating their public sphere and altering the basic character of French culture" (Beale, *The Modernist Enterprise,* 57, 46, 14–15).

68. Beale, *The Modernist Enterprise,* esp. chap. 1.

69. A. Coulonge, ". . . En médecine et pharmacie: madame se meurt . . . madame ne veut pas mourir," *La publicité de France,* no. 2 (November 15, 1923): 19.

70. Ibid., 30.

71. Ibid.

72. Ibid., 30–32.

73. R. Lieters, "Quelques idées sur les étalages des pharmaciens," *La publicité de France,* no. 8 (May 15, 1924): 51–54.

74. Ibid.

75. "Pour faire des affaires dans la coiffure," *La coiffure de Paris: Revue professionnelle, illustrée, artistique, littéraire, scientifique* 187 (September 1925): 30–31. This percentage varied depending on the type of salon and its clientele.

76. Robert Sauleau, "L'étalage," *La coiffure de Paris: Revue professionnelle, illustrée, artistique, littéraire, scientifique* 204 (February 10, 1927): 20.

77. Ibid. He advised coiffures to sell their products at an advertised price and to prominently list prices for both goods and services in a "table of prices based on the American model."

78. Here I identify the coiffure as masculine and the customer as feminine because that is how contributors to the journal identified them.

79. Arvet-Thouvet, "Peut-on être un bon commerçant," *La coiffure de Paris: Revue professionnelle, illustrée, artistique, littéraire, scientifique,* no. 246 (August 1930): 35, 37.

80. Zdatny, *Fashion, Work, and Politics,* 97.

81. Arvet-Thouvet, "Peut-on être un bon commerçant," 35.

82. The respected Parisian hairstylist and innovator Emile Long was distressed that fashionable women, as well as women of the middle and working classes, were adopting the "horrible fashion" in "epidemic proportions." The immediate situation appeared so dire, in fact, that the trade journal *La coiffure de Paris* offered a five-thousand-franc award to any stylist who could create a new style that might compete with or overtake the bob (Zdatny, *Fashion, Work, and Politics*, 62–65).

83. A. Pesch, "La manicurie," *La coiffure de Paris: Revue professionnelle illustrée. artistique, littéraire, scientifique* 196 (June 10, 1926): 25; A. Pesch, "Le massage facial et les soins esthétiques," *La coiffure de Paris: Revue professionnelle illustrée. artistique, littéraire, scientifique* 201 (November 10, 1926): 31; A. S. "Les soins de beauté chez le coiffeur," *La coiffure de Paris: Revue professionnelle illustrée. artistique, littéraire, scientifique* 218 (April 1, 1928): 19.

84. Antoine Crème Astringent ad, *Vogue*, 1927 (multiple issues).

85. Zdatny, *Fashion, Work, and Politics*, 58.

86. Arvet-Thouvet, "La parfumerie aux coiffeurs? L'exemple de Dusseldorf," *La coiffure de Paris: Revue professionnelle, illustrée, artistique, littéraire, scientifique* (December 1936): 19.

87. Arvet-Thouvet, "Le parfumeur 'sert' mais le coiffeur 'offer,'" *La coiffure de Paris: Revue professionnelle, illustrée, artistique, littéraire, scientifique* (February 1938): 15.

88. M. de Presle, "Sauvez vous-mêmes vos finances," *La coiffure de Paris: Revue professionnelle, illustrée, artistique, littéraire, scientifique* (March 1938): 20.

89. Gabriel Fau, "Pourquoi ne deviendrions-nous pas des Coiffeurs-Parfumeurs?" *La coiffure de Paris: Revue professionnelle, illustrée, artistique, littéraire, scientifique* (July 1936): 28.

90. Ibid.

91. M. de Presle, "Sauvez vous-mêmes vos finances," *La coiffure de Paris: Revue professionnelle, illustrée, artistique, littéraire, scientifique* (March 1938): 20.

92. "Pour vendre 'plus' vendons de la 'qualité,'" *La coiffure de Paris: Revue professionnelle, illustrée, artistique, littéraire, scientifique* (December 1938): 21–22.

93. Madeleine Ray, *Notre santé et notre charme: L'hygiène moderne et les soins délicats dont la pratique met en valeur la grâce feminine* (Paris: Éditions Gautier-Languereau, 1932). Similar manuals from the period include Maxime Curtin, *Jeunesse et beauté. Vitalité. Ce qui l'augmente. Ce qui la diminue* (Paris: Aberg pratique d'hygiène moderne, 1921); Delarue-Mardrus, *Embellissez-vous;* Eugène Marsan, *Pour habiller éliant où le nouveau secret des dames* (Paris: A. Liege, 1927); and Jeanne Myrtile, *Pour être toujours belle* (Paris: France-éditions, 1922).

94. Ray, *Notre santé et notre charme*, 64, 77–78.

95. Ibid., 154–55.

96. Ibid., 158–60. I have condensed the steps here, highlighting main points and eliminating the author's elaborations.

97. Alfred A. Bitterlin, *L'art de faire sa beauté* (Paris: Éditions Drouin, 1925), 10–11.

98. Ibid., 16.

99. Ibid., 27.

100. Ibid., 41.

101. Sylvie, *Comment je fais ma beauté.*

102. Françose Arnoux, "La clarté d'un beau visage," *Femina*, Autumn 1931.

103. "La science du chimiste au service de la beauté," *Femina*, February 1932, 32–33.

104. "A la conquete d'une nouvelle jeunesse," *Vogue,* April 1, 1923, 41–42, 62.

105. Marie-Claire Duchenne, "La science de la beauté : S'enrichit chaque jour de découvertes nouvelles," *Femina,* November 1932, 21–22.

106. Claude Malays, "Petite bréviaire de la beauté: Ce que toute femme doit faire pour être agréable à regarder," *Femina,* August 1934, 30–31.

107. "Know Your Evening Makeup," *Votre Beauté,* special issue, Christmas 1936, 67–68.

108. "Michel Arbaud, "Le maquillage individual: Comment établir le vôtre sans erreur possible," *Votre beauté,* October 1937, 27–30.

109. Ibid., 27.

110. Ibid., 30.

111. *Votre beauté,* November 1937, 27–29.

112. Ibid., 27. I interpret "certain" as "desired."

113. By 1936, *Votre beauté* (by my own count) was publishing around eighty reader letters per issue and devoting at least seven pages of the magazine to reader concerns.

114. "Budgets de Beauté," *Votre beauté,* April 1936, 1–2, 5. Starting in the 1930s, *Votre beauté* also published articles that specifically targeted the "working woman."

115. "In that time of crisis," she explained, "women really needed their beauty. One had to be beautiful even when one had few new clothes and fewer trinkets to adorn them. One had also to be young, or seem to be, to find a job. Keeping one's charm was the first concern among all women" (Odette Arnaud, "Métiers féminins—beauté, mon beau souci," *Miroir du monde,* January 26, 1935, 91). I thank Rebecca Scales for bringing this article to my attention.

116. Léon-Martin, *L'industrie de la beauté* (Paris: Éditions des Portiques, 1930), 30–31.

CONCLUSION

1. Jacques Dourdin, *Étude du marche de la parfumerie* (Paris: Commission Intersyndicale de la Parfumerie, 1949).

2. Ibid., 17.

3. Ibid., 32–33.

4. Pougy, *My Blue Notebooks,* 102.

5. Clara Malraux, *Memoirs,* trans. Patrick O'Brian (New York: Farrar, Straus and Giroux, 1967), 315.

6. Ibid., 17–20.

7. Corbin, *The Foul and the Fragrant;* Vigarello, *Concepts of Cleanliness.*

8. Butler, "Performative Acts," 271.

9. Liz Conor, *The Spectacular Modern Woman: Feminine Visibility in the 1920s* (Bloomington: Indiana University Press, 2004), 2, 6, 7.

10. Beauvoir, *The Second Sex,* 595.

11. Ibid., 270–71.

12. Ibid., 594.

13. N. C. Baker, *The Beauty Trap* (New York: Franklin Watts, 1984); Fenja Gunn, *The Artificial Face: A History of Cosmetics* (New York: Hippocrene, 1973); Naomi Wolf, *The Beauty Myth: How Images of Beauty Are Used Against Women* (New York: William Morrow, 1991).

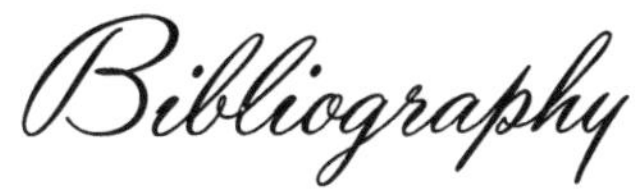

Bibliography

ARCHIVAL MATERIALS

Archives nationales de France
Series AZ: Department Store Dossier, late nineteenth/early twentieth centuries
Series AQ: Dossier Bon Marché; Dossier Printemps; Dossier Aux Dames de France
Bibliothèque de l'arsenal: Fonds Rondel
Bibliothèque Forney: Catalogue Commericaux; Fonds Grands Magasins; Fonds iconographique
Bibliothèque historique de la Ville de Paris
4Z 204: Agenda de la Place Clichy, 1911–1912
4Z 211: Agenda de la Maison des Magasins du Louvre, 1879–1930
4Z 287: Agenda des Galeries Lafayettes, 1913
Bibliothèque Marguerite Durand: Dossier Beauté; Dossier Josephine Baker

PRIMARY SOURCES

Periodicals

Archives de la droguerie pharmaceutique de l'herboristerie, des produits et spécialités pharmaceutiques, accessoires, etc . . . Journal indépendant paraissant tous les mois (1933–1938)
Beauté (1929–1932)
La coiffure de Paris: Revue professionnelle, illustrée, artistique, littéraire, scientifique (1909–1939)
La coiffure et les modes/Beauté-coiffeur-mode/Votre beauté (1927–1940)
Commerce et industrie (1907–1914)
Etalages et présentation (1932–1936)
Femina (1901–1957)
Illustration (1924)

Monsieur, Revue des élégances (1920–1922)
La parfumerie moderne: Revue scientifique et de défense professionnelle... (1909–1911)
La publicité de France (1923–1924)
La vie de Paris (1898–1899)
Vogue (édition française) (1920–1939)

Books and Articles

André-Valdès. *Encyclopédie illustrée des élégances: Hygiène de la beauté.* Paris: Librairie Marpon et Flammarion, 1892.

Arvet-Thouvet. "Le parfumeur 'sert' mais le coiffeur 'offer.'" *La coiffure de Paris: Revue professionnelle, illustrée, artistique, littéraire, scientifique* (February 1938): 15.

——. "La perfumerie aux coiffeurs? L'exemple de Dusseldorf." *La coiffure de Paris: Revue professionnelle, illustrée, artistique, littéraire, scientifique* (December 1936): 19.

——. "Peut-on être un bon commerçant." *La coiffure de Paris: Revue professionnelle, illustrée, artistique, littéraire, scientifique* 246 (August 1930): 35, 37.

Aux femmes chretiennes: Le scandale de la mode. Besançon: Imprimerie de l'est, 1923.

Baudelaire, Charles. *The Painter of Modern Life.* Translated by Jonathan Mayne. New York: Phaidon, 1964.

——. *Le peintre de la vie moderne.* 1863. www.uniduisburg.de/lyriktheorie/1863_baudelaire.com.

Bitterlin, Alfred A. *L'art de faire sa beauté.* Paris: Éditions Drouin, 1925.

Boulenger, Jacques. "La femme moderne: Devant le feu." *Illustration,* December 6, 1924.

Cavalieri, Lina. *My Secrets of Beauty.* New York: Circulation Syndicate, 1914.

Colette, Sidonie-Gabrielle. *Belles Saison: A Colette Scrapbook.* Compiled by Robert Phelps. Translated by Matthew Ward. New York: Farrar, Straus and Giroux, 1983.

——. *Chéri.* Paris: Arthème Fayard, 1920.

——. *"Chéri" and "The Last of Chéri."* Trans. Roger Senhouse. New York: Penguin, 1977.

——. *The Collected Stories of Colette.* Edited by Robert Phelps. Translated by Matthew Ward, Antonia White, and Anne-Marie Callimach. New York: Farrar, Straus and Giroux, 1983.

——. "Fards, poudres, parfums." *Femina,* November 1927, 23.

——. *Letters from Colette.* Selected and translated by Robert Phelps. New York: Farrar, Straus and Giroux, 1980.

——. *Lettres à Hélène Picard.* Edited by Charles Pichois. Paris: Flammarion, 1988.

——. *Lettres de la vagabonde.* Edited by Claude Pichoise and R. Forbin. Paris: Flammarion, 1961.

——. *Mes apprentissages.* Translated by Helen Beauclerk. New York: Farrar, Straus and Giroux, 1957.

——. *The Shackle.* Translated by Antonia White. New York: Farrar, Straus and Giroux, 1964.

——. *The Vagabond.* Translated by Enid McLeod. New York: Penguin, 1960.

——. *La vagabonde.* Paris: Librairie Paul Ollendorff, 1910.

Coulonge, A. "... En médecine et pharmacie: Madame se meurt... madame ne veut pas mourir." *La publicité de France,* no. 2 (November 15, 1923).

——. "... En médecine et pharmacie vos étalages." *La publicité de France,* no. 4 (January 1924).

Curtin, Maxime. *Jeunesse et beauté. Vitalité. Ce qui l'augmente. Ce qui la diminue.* Paris: Aberg pratique d'hygiène moderne, 1921.

Delarue-Mardrus, Lucie. *Embellissez-vous!* Paris: Éditions de France, 1926.

Dhur, Jacques. "Coiffeurs et pharmaciens." *La parfumerie moderne,* no. 1 (January 1910): 88–89.

Dumont, Arsène. *Dépopulation et civilisation; Étude démographique.* Paris: Lecrosnier et Babé, 1890.

Fau, Gabriel. "Pourquoi ne deviendrions-nous pas des Coiffeurs-Parfumeurs?" *La coiffure de Paris: Revue professionnelle, illustrée, artistique, littéraire, scientifique* (July 1936): 28.

Freulon, Robert. *Notes sur la publicité.* Paris, 1923.

Goublet, Juliette. "Colette et la beauté." *Beauté-coiffure-mode/Votre beauté,* June 1932, 11

Goudeket, Maurice. *Close to Colette.* Trans. Enid McLeod. London: Secker and Warburg, 1957.

Langrand, André. Response to Jacques Dhur. *La parfumerie moderne,* no. 1 (January 1910).

Lapin, Jules. "Nos conférences: La psychologie dans les affaires." *Commerce et industrie,* no. 22 (March 20, 1909): 100–105.

Léon-Martin, Louis. *L'industrie de la beauté.* Paris: Éditions des Portiques, 1930.

Lieters, R. "Quelques idées sur les étalages des pharmaciens." *La publicité de France,* no. 8 (May 15, 1924): 51–54.

Malraux, Clara. *Le bruit de nos pas III: Les Combats et les Jeux.* Paris: Éditions Bernard Grasset, 1969.

——. *Memoirs.* Translated by Patrick O'Brian. New York: Farrar, Straus and Giroux, 1967.

Marrin, Dr. P. *La beauté chez l'homme et chez la femme: Les moyens de l'acquérir, de la conserver, de l'augmenter.* Paris: Ernest Kolb, 1905.

Marsan, Eugène. *Pour habiller eliante éliante? Ou le nouveau secret des dames.* Paris: A. Liege, 1927.

Ministère du commerce, de l'industrie des postes et des Ttlégraphes. *Exposition universelle internationale de 1900: Rapports du Jury International, Groupe XVI—*

Économique sociale.—Hygiène—Assistance publique. Paris: Imprimerie Nationale, 1900.

Monin, Ernest. *Hygiène et médicine féminines: Secrets de santé et de beauté.* Paris, 1901.

Myrtile, Jeanne. *Pour être toujours belle.* Paris: France-éditions, 1922.

Norville, Comtesse de. *Les coulisses de la beauté: Comment la femme séduit.* Paris: S. Ampleman, 1895.

Otera, Caroline. *My Story.* London: A. M. Philpot, 1927.

Parent-Duchaelet, A.J.B. *De la prostitution dans la ville de Paris, considérée sous le rapport de l'hygiène publique, de la morale et de l'administration . . .* Paris: J. B. Baillière; New York: H. Baillière, 1857.

Payot, Dr. Nadia Grégoire. *Être belle.* Paris: Presses universitaires de France, 1933.

Piesse, Septimus. *Histoire des parfums et hygiène de la toilette.* Paris: Librairie J-B Ballire et Fils, 1905.

Pougy, Liane de. *My Blue Notebooks: The Intimate Journal of Paris's Most Beautiful and Notorious Courtesan.* New York: Tarcher/Putnam, 1979.

"Pour faire des affaires dans la coiffure." *La coiffure de Paris: Revue professionnelle, illustrée, artistique, littéraire, scientifique* 187 (September 1925): 30–31.

"Pour vendre 'plus', vendons de la 'qualité.'" *La coiffure de Paris: Revue professionnelle, illustrée, artistique, littéraire, scientifique* (December 1938): 21–22.

Presle, M. de. "Sauvez vous-mêmes vos finances." *La coiffure de Paris: Revue professionnelle, illustrée, artistique, littéraire, scientifique* (March 1938): 20.

Pougy, Liane de. *My Blue Notebooks: The Intimate Journal of Paris's Most Beautiful and Notorious Courtesan.* Translated by Diana Athill. New York: Penguin Putnam, 1979.

Ray, Madeleine. *Notre santé et notre charme: L'hygiène moderne et les soins délicats dont la pratique met en valeur la grâce feminine.* Paris: Éditions Gautier-Languereau, 1932.

Ris-Paquot. *Hygiène, médicine, parfumerie, pharmacie.* Paris: Librairie Renouard, 1894.

Rousseau, Jean-Jacques. "Discourse on the Origin and Foundations of Inequality among Men or Second Discourse." In *Rousseau, the Discourses and Other Writings,* edited by Victor Gourevitch. Cambridge: Cambridge University Press, 1997.

——. Émile. Translated by Barbara Foxley. London: Dent and Dutton, 1963.

——. "Letter to Alembert on the Theater." In *Letter to d'Alembert and Writings for the Theater,* edited by and translated by Allan Bloom, Charles Butterworth, and Christopher Kelly. Hanover, N.H.: University Press of New England, 2004.

Saint-Merry, Pol de. *Petite bibliothèque du coeur.* Paris: H. Geoffroy, 1898.

Sauleau, Robert. "L'étalage." *La coiffure de Paris: Revue professionnelle, illustrée, artistique, littéraire, scientifique* 204 (February 10, 1927): 20.

Schultz, Doctoresse M. *Hygiène générale de la femme. alimentation—vêtements—soins corporels d'après l'enseignement et la pratique du Docteur Auvard.* Paris: Octave Doin, 1903.

Sylvie. *Comment je fais ma beauté.* Paris: Éditions de "Femme de France," 1937.

Tramar, Comtesse de. *A la conquête du bonheur!* Paris: A. Maloine, 1912.

——. *Le bréviaire de la femme: Pratiques secrets de la beauté.* Paris: Victor-Havard, 1903.

Uzanne, Octave. *Fashion in Paris: The Various Phases of Feminine Taste and Aesthetics from 1797 to 1897.* Translated by Lady Mary Loyd. London: Heinemann; New York: Scribner's Sons, 1898.

Waleffe, Maurice de. *Quand Paris était un paradis, mémoires, 1900–1939.* Paris: Société des éditions Denoël, 1947.

Zola, Émile. *Nana.* Paris: G. Charpentier, 1888.

——. *Nana.* Translated by Douglas Parmée. New York: Oxford University Press, 1992.

——. "Une nouvelle manière en peinture: Édouard Manet." *Revue du dix-neuvième siècle,* January 1, 1867.

SECONDARY SOURCES

Abelson, Elaine S. *When Ladies Go A-Thieving: Middle-Class Shoplifters in the Victorian Department Store.* New York: Oxford University Press, 1990.

Abescat, Bruno. *La saga des Bettencourt, L'Oréal: Une fortune française.* Paris: Plon, 2002.

Acampo, Elinor. *Gender and the Politics of Social Reform in France, 1870–1914.* Baltimore: Johns Hopkins University Press, 1995.

Adorno, Theodor W., and Max Horkheimer. "The Culture Industry: Enlightenment as Mass Deception." In *Dialectic of Enlightenment,* by Adorno and Horkheimer. London: Verso, 1979.

Apter, Emily. "Cabinet Secret: Fetishism, Prostitution, and the Fin-de-Siècle Interior." *Assemblage,* no. 9 (June 1989).

Armstrong, Carol. *Manet Manette.* New Haven: Yale University Press, 2002.

Arnold, Rebecca. *Fashion, Desire, and Anxiety: Image and Morality in the Twentieth Century.* New Brunswick, N.J.: Rutgers University Press, 2001.

Baker, Keith. "Defining the Public Sphere in Eighteenth-Century France: Variations of a Theme by Habermas." In *Habermas and the Public Sphere,* edited by Craig Calhoun. Cambridge: MIT Press, 1992.

Baker, N. C. *The Beauty Trap.* New York: Franklin Watts, 1984.

Ballerino Cohen, Colleen, Richard Wilk, and Beverly Stoeltje, eds. *Beauty Queens on the Global Stage: Gender, Contests, and Power.* London: Routledge, 1996.

Banner, Lois. *American Beauty.* Chicago: University of Chicago Press, 1984.

Bard, Christine. *Les garçonnes: Modes et fantasmes des années folles.* Paris: Flammarion, 1998.

Barillé, Elisabeth. *Coty: Parfumeur et visionnaire.* Paris: Éditions Assouline, 1995.

Barthel, Diane. *Putting on Appearances: Gender and Advertising.* Philadelphia: Temple University Press, 1988.

Bartky, Sandra Lee. *Femininity and Domination.* New York: Routledge, 1990.

Baudrillard, Jean. *Seduction.* New York: St. Martin's Press, 1990.

——. *Selected Writings.* Stanford, Calif.: Stanford University Press, 1970.

Beale, Marjorie A. *The Modernist Enterprise: French Elites and the Threat of Modernity, 1900–1940.* Stanford: Stanford University Press, 1999.

Beauvoir, Simone de. *The Second Sex.* New York: Vintage, 1952.

Beizer, Janet L. "Uncovering Nana: The Courtesan's New Clothes." *L'esprit créateur* 25, no. 2 (1985): 45–56.

Beken, Micheline van der. *Zola, le-dessous des femmes.* Brussels: Le cri édition, 2000.

Bergeron, Louis. *Les industries du luxe en France.* Paris: Éditions Odile Jacob, 1998.

Berlanstein, Lenard. *Daughters of Eve: A Cultural History of French Theater Women from the Old Regime to the Fin de Siècle.* Cambridge: Harvard University Press, 2004.

——. "Historicizing and Gendering Celebrity Culture: Famous Women in Nineteenth-Century France." *Journal of Women's History* 16, no. 4 (Winter 2004): 65–91.

——. "Selling Modern Femininity: *Femina,* a Forgotten Feminist Publishing Success in Belle Epoque France." *French Historical Studies* 30, no. 4 (Fall 2007): 623–49.

Bernheimer, Charles. *Figures of Ill-Repute: Representing Prostitution in Nineteenth-Century France.* Durham, N.C., Duke University Press, 1997.

——. "Manet's Olympia: The Figuration of Scandal." *Poetics Today* 10, no. 2 (Summer 1989): 255–77.

Berry, Francesca. "Designing the Reader's Interior: Subjectivity and the Woman's Magazine in Early Twentieth-Century France." *Journal of Design History* 18, no. 1 (2005): 61–79.

Berry, Sarah. *Screen Style: Fashion and Femininity in 1930s Hollywood.* Minneapolis: University of Minnesota Press, 2000.

Best, Victoria. *Critical Subjectivities: Identity and Narrative in the Work of Colette and Marguerite Duras.* Bern: Peter Lang, 2000.

Bonal, Gérard, and Frédéric Maget, eds. *Colette journaliste: Chroniques et reportages 1893–1955.* Paris: Éditions seuil, 2010.

Bonzon, Thierry. "The Labour Market and Industrial Mobilization, 1915–1917." In *Capital Cities at War: Paris, London, Berlin, 1914–1919,* edited by Jay Winter and Jean-Louis Robert. Cambridge: Cambridge University Press, 1997.

Bourdieu, Pierre. *Distinction A Social Critique of the Judgment of Taste.* Translated by Richard Nice. Cambridge: Harvard University Press, 1984.

Brooks, Peter. "Storied Bodies, or Nana at Last Unveil'd." *Critical Inquiry* 16, no. 1 (Autumn 1989): 1–32.

Brownmiller, S. *Femininity.* New York: Linden, 1984.

Butler, Judith. *Gender Trouble: Feminism and the Subversion of Identity.* New York: Routledge, 2008.

———. "Performative Acts and Gender Constitution: An Essay in Phenomenology and Feminist Theory." In *Performing Feminisms: Feminist Critical Theory and the Theatre,* edited by Sue Ellen Case. Baltimore: Johns Hopkins University Press, 1990.

Canning, Kathleen. *Gender History in Practice: Historical Perspectives on Bodies, Class, and Citizenship.* Ithaca, N.Y.: Cornell University Press, 2006.

Certeau, Michel de. *The Practice of Everyday Life.* Translated by Steven Rendall. Berkeley: University of California Press, 1984.

Chadwick, Whitney, and Tirza True Latimer, eds. *The Modern Woman Revisited: Paris between the Wars.* New Brunswick, N.J.: Rutgers University Press, 2003.

Cheng, Anne Anlin. "Wounded Beauty: An Exploratory Essay on Race, Feminism, and the Aesthetic Question." *Tulsa Studies in Women's Literature* 19, no. 2 (Autumn 2000): 191–217.

Chenut, Helen. *The Fabric of Gender: Working-Class Culture in Third Republic France.* State College: Pennsylvania State University Press, 2006.

Chernin, K. *Womansize: The Tyranny of Slenderness.* London: Women's Press, 1983.

Chevrel, Claudine, and Béatrice Cornet, eds. *Grain de beauté: Un siècle de beauté par la publicité.* Paris: Somogy éditions d'art, Bibliothèque Forney, 1993.

Clark, Anna. *Desire: A History of European Sexuality.* New York: Routledge, 2008.

Clark, Linda. "Bringing Feminine Qualities in the Public Sphere: The Third Republic's Appointment of Female Inspectors." In *Gender and the Politics of Social Reform in France, 1870–1914,* edited by Eleanor Acampo. Baltimore: Johns Hopkins University Press, 1995.

Clark, T. J. *The Painting of Modern Life: Paris in the Art of Manet and His Followers.* Rev. ed. Princeton, N.J.: Princeton University Press, 1984.

Cole, Joshua. *The Power of Large Numbers: Population, Politics, and Gender in Nineteenth-Century France.* Ithaca, N.Y.: Cornell University Press, 2000.

Collado, Melanie E. *Colette, Lucie-Delarue-Mardrus, Marcelle Tinayre: Émancipation et résignation.* Paris: Harmattan, 2003.

Comisky, Carolyn. "Cosmetic Surgery in Paris in 1926: The Case of the Amputated Leg." *Journal of Women's History* 16, no. 3 (Fall 2004): 30–54.

Conway, Kelly. *Chanteuse in the City: The Realist Singer in French Film.* Berkeley: University of California Press, 2004.

Corbin, Alain. *Le miasme et la jonquille: L'odorat et l'imaginaire social XVIIIe–XIXe siècles.* Paris: Aubier Montaigne, 1982.

———. *Women for Hire: Prostitution and Sexuality in France after 1850.* Cambridge: Harvard University Press, 1990.

Coward, R. *Female Desire: Women's Sexuality Today.* London: Paladin, 1984.

Crossick, Geoffrey, and Serge Jaumain, eds. *Cathedrals of Consumption: The European Department Store, 1850–1939.* London: Ashgate, 1999.

Cummins, Laurel. *Colette and the Conquest of Self.* Birmingham, Ala.: Summa, 2005.
Dalle, François. *L'aventure L'Oréal.* Paris: Jacob, 2001.
Darrow, Margaret H. *French Women and the First World War: War Stories of the Home Front.* Oxford: Berg, 2000.
Davey, Lynda. "La croquese d'hommes: Images de la protituée chez Flaubert, Zola, et Maupassant." *Romantisme* 17, no. 58 (1987): 59–66.
David, Delphine. *La distribution de parfums et produits de beauté: Quelle redistribution des cartes?* Institut Xerfi, Conjuncture secteurs d'entreprise & recherches financières. April 1997.
Debue-Barazer, Christine. "Le médicament 1803–1940." March 2003. www.ordre.pharmacien.fr, pp. 1–5, Documents de référence—Histoire et art pharmaceutique.
De Courtivron, Isabelle. "'Never Admit!': Colette and the Freedom of Paradox." In *The Modern Woman Revisited: Paris between the Wars,* edited by Whitney Chadwick and Tirza True Latimer, 55–64. New Brunswick, N.J.: Rutgers University Press, 2003.
De Grazia, Victoria. *The Sex of Things: Gender and Consumption in Historical Perspective.* With Ellen Furlough. Berkeley: University of California Press, 1996.
Delbourg-Delphis, Marylène. *Le chic et le look: Histoire de la mode feminine et des moeurs de 1850 à nos jours.* Paris: Hachette, 1981.
Desan, Suzanne. *The Family on Trial in the Revolutionary France.* Berkeley: University of California Press, 2004.
Ellis, Aytoun. *The Essence of Beauty: A History of Perfume and Cosmetics.* London: Secker and Warburg, 1960.
Ellis, Jack D. *The Physician-Legislators of France: Medicine and Politics in the Early Third Republic, 1870–1914.* Cambridge: Cambridge University Press, 1990.
Featherstone, Mike. "The Body in Consumer Culture." In *The Body: Social Process and Cultural Theory,* edited by Featherstone, Mike Hepworth, and Bryan S. Turner, 170–96. London: Sage, 1991.
Felman, Shoshana. "Rereading Femininity." *Yale French Studies,* no. 62 (1981): 19–44.
Finkelstein, J. *The Fashioned Self.* Oxford: Polity, 1991.
Fischer, Lucy. *Designing Women: Cinema, Art Deco, and the Female Form.* New York: Columbia University Press, 2003.
Fouassier, Eric. "Le cadre général de la loi du 21 Germinal An XI." March 2003. www.ordre.pharmacien.fr, Documents de référence—Histoire et art pharmaceutique.
Foucault, Michel. *Discipline and Punish: The Birth of the Prison.* New York: Vintage, 1977.
——. *The History of Sexuality: Volume One: An Introduction.* New York: Vintage, 1990.
Francis, Claude, and Fernande Gontier. *Creating Colette.* Vol. 2, *From Baroness to Woman of Letters, 1912–1954.* South Royalton, Vt.: Steerforth, 1999.
Freadman, Ann. "Laurel Cummins, Colette and the Conquest of Self." *French Studies* 61, no. 1 (2007): 118–19.

Freud, Sigmund. *Three Essays on the Theory of Sexuality.* Trans. James Strachey. New York: Basic, 2000.

Frost, Robert. "Machine Liberation: Inventing Housewives and Home Appliances in InterwarFrance." *French Historical Studies* 18, no. 1 (Spring 1993): 109–30.

Fryer, Paul, and Olga Usova. *Lina Cavalieri: The Life of Opera's Greatest Beauty, 1874–1944.* Jefferson, N.C.: McFarland, 2004.

Furlough, Ellen. *Consumer Cooperation in France: The Politics of Consumption, 1834–1930.* Ithaca, N.Y.: Cornell University Press, 1991.

———. "Selling the American Way in Interwar France: *Prix Uniques* and the *Salons des Arts Menagers* in Interwar France. *Journal of Social History* 26, no. 3 (Spring 1993): 491–519.

Gagnier, Regina. *Subjectivities: A History of Self-Representation in Britain, 1832–1920.* New York: Oxford University Press, 1991.

Gallagher, Catherine, and Thomas Laqueur, eds. *The Making of the Modern Body: Sexuality and Society in the Nineteenth Century.* Berkeley: University of California Press, 1987.

Gay, Peter. *The Education of the Senses.* Vol. 1 of *The Bourgeois Experience: Victoria to Freud.* New York: Oxford University Press, 1984.

———. *Pleasure Wars.* Vol. 5 of *The Bourgeois Experience: Victoria to Freud.* New York: Norton, 1998.

Gerbord, Paul. "Les coiffeurs en France (1800–1950)." *Le mouvement social,* no. 14 (January–March 1981): 71–84.

Ghozland, F., and J-P Forestier. *Cosmétiques. être et paraître.* Milan: Éditions Milan, 1987.

Goldstein, Jan. "Foucault among the Sociologists: The "Disciplines" and the History of the Professions." *History and Theory* 23, no. 2 (May 1984): 170–92.

Goodman, Dena. "Public Sphere and Private Life: Toward a Synthesis of Current Historiographical Approaches to the Old Regime." *History and Theory* 31, no. 1 (1992): 1–20.

Grayzel, Susan. *Women's Identities at War: Gender, Motherhood, and Politics in Britain and France during the First World War.* Chapel Hill: University of North Carolina Press, 1999.

Greenhalgh, Paul. *Ephemeral Vistas: The Expositons Universelles, Great Exhibitions, and World's Fairs, 1851–1939.* New York: Manchester University Press, 1988.

Gundle, Stephen. *Glamour: A History.* New York: Oxford University Press, 2008.

Gunn, Fenja. *The Artificial Face: A History of Cosmetics.* New York: Hippocrene, 1973.

Haedrich, Marcel. *Coco Chanel: Her Life, Her Secrets.* Boston: Little, Brown, 1972.

Harris, Gerry. "Regarding History: Some Narratives Concerning the Café-concert, Le Music Hall, and the Feminist Academic." *Drama Review* 40, no. 4 (Winter 1996): 70–84.

Harrow, Susan. *Zola, the Body Modern: Pressures and Prospects of Representation.* London: Legenda, 2010.

Harsin, Jill. *Policing Prostitution in Nineteenth-Century Paris.* Princeton, N.J.: Princeton University Press, 1985.

Hause, Steven C. "More Minerva than Mars: The French Women's Rights Campaign and the First World War." In *Behind the Lines: Gender and the Two World Wars,* edited by Margaret Randolph Higonnet, Jane Jenson, Sonya Michel, and Margaret Collings Weitz, 99–113. New Haven: Yale University Press, 1987.

Hautefort, Jean-Michel. *Parfumerie-cosmétique: Les nouveaux enjeux.* Paris: Eurostaf–Les echos études, 2000.

Hiner, Susan. *Accessories to Modernity: Fashion and the Feminine in Nineteenth-Century France.* State College: University of Pennsylvania Press, 2010.

Hultquist, Clark. "The Price of Dreams: A History of Advertising in France, 1927–1968." Ph.D. diss., Ohio State University, 1996.

Hunt, Lynn. *The Family Romance of the French Revolution.* Berkeley: University of California Press, 1992.

Israel, Lee. *Estée Lauder: Beyond the Magic.* New York: Macmillan, 1985.

Jay, Martin. *Downcast Eyes: The Denigration of Vision in Twentieth-Century French Thought.* Berkeley: University of California Press, 1993.

Jones, Jennifer. "Repackaging Rousseau: Femininity and Fashion in Old Regime France." *French Historical Studies* 18, no. 4 (Autumn 1994): 939–67.

——. *Sexing la Mode: Gender, Fashion, and Commercial Culture in Old Regime France.* New York: Berg, 2004.

Julièr, Irène. "Le maquillage, pratiques, discours, et interprétations." Ph.D. diss., Paris VII, 1989.

Koehn, Nancy. "Estée Lauder, Self-Definition and the Modern Cosmetics Market." In *Beauty and Business: Commerce, Gender, and Culture in Modern America,* edited by Philip Scranton, 217–51. New York: Routledge, 2001.

Krumm, Pascale. "Nana maternelle: oxymore?" *French Review* 69, no. 2 (December 1995): 217–28.

Kwass, Michael. "Big Hair: A Wig History of Consumption in Eighteenth-Century France." *American Historical Review* 111, no. 3 (June 2006): 631–59.

Laqueur, Thomas. *Making Sex: Body and Gender from the Greeks to Freud.* Cambridge: Harvard University Press, 1990.

——. "Orgasm, Generation, and the Politics of Reproductive Biology." In "The Making of the Modern Body: Sexuality and Society in the Nineteenth Century," special issue, *Representations* 14 (Spring 1986): 1–41.

Leach, William. "Strategists of Display and the Production of Desire." In *Consuming Visions: Accumulation and Display of Goods in America, 1880–1920,* edited by Simon J. Bronner, 99–132. New York: Norton, 1989.

Lucey, Michael. *Never Say I: Sexuality and the First Person in Colette, Gide, and Proust.* Durham, N.C.: Duke University Press, 2006.

Lury, Celia. *Consumer Culture.* New Brunswick, N.J.: Rutgers University Press, 1996.

Maier, Charles S. "Between Taylorism and Technocracy: European Ideologies and the Vision of Industrial Productivity in the 1920s." *Journal of Contemporary History* 5, no. 2 (1970): 27–61.

Maisonneuve, Jean, and Marilou Bruchon-Schweitzer. *Le corps et la beauté.* Paris: Presses Universitaires de France, 1999.

Manko, Katina L. "A Depression Proof Business Strategy: The California Perfume Company's Motivational Literature." In *Beauty and Business: Commerce, Gender, and Culture in Modern America,* edited by Philip Scranton, 142–68. New York: Routledge, 2001.

Martin, Marc. "Structures de societé et consciences rebelles: Les resistances à la publicité dans la France de l'entre-deux guerres." *Le mouvement sociale,* no. 146 (January–March 1989): 27–48.

Martin, Morag. "Consuming Beauty: The Commerce of Cosmetics in France, 1750–1800." Ph.D. diss., University of California, Irvine, 1999.

———. *Selling Beauty: Cosmetics, Commerce, and French Society, 1750–1830.* Baltimore: Johns Hopkins University Press, 2009.

Marwick, Arthur. *Beauty in History: Society, Politics, and Personal Appearance c. 1500 to the Present.* London: Thames and Hudson, 1985.

McMillan, James F. *France and Women 1789–1914: Gender, Society and Politics.* London: Routledge, 2000.

Menon, Elizabeth K. *Evil by Design: The Creation and Marketing of the Femme Fatale.* Urbana: University of Illinois Press, 2006.

Mesch, Rachel. *Having It All in the Belle Epoque: How French Women's Magazines Invented the Modern Woman.* Stanford, Calif.: Stanford University Press, 2013.

Miller, Michael. *Au Bon Marché: Bourgeois Culture and the Department Store, 1869–1920.* Princeton, N.J.: Princeton University Press, 1981.

Modern Girl Around the World Research Group. *The Modern Girl Around the World: Consumption, Modernity, and Globalization.* Edited by Alys Eve Weinbaum, *Lynn M. Thomas, Priti Ramamurthy, Uta G. Poiger,* and *Madeleine Yue Dong.* Durham, N.C.: Duke University Press, 2008.

———. "The Modern Girl Around the World: A Research Agenda and Preliminary Findings." *Gender and History* 17, no. 3 (August 2005): 245–94.

Modleski, T., ed. *Studies in Entertainment.* Bloomington: Indiana University Press, 1986.

Morck, Randall K., ed. *A History of Corporate Governance around the World: Family Business Groups and Professional Managers.* Chicago: University of Chicago Press, 2005.

Mulvey, Laura. *Visual and Other Pleasures.* London: Routledge, 1984.

Nead, Lynda. *The Female Nude: Art, Obscenity, and Sexuality.* London: Routledge, 1992.

Negrin, Llewellyn. "The Self as Image: A Critical Appraisal of Postmodern Theories of Fashion." *Theory, Culture & Society* 163, no. 3 (1999): 99–118.

Nolan, Mary. *Visions of Modernity: American Business and the Modernization of Germany.* New York: Oxford University Press, 1994.

Nye, Robert. *Crime, Madness, and Politics in Modern France: The Medical Concept of National Decline.* Princeton, N.J.: Princeton University Press, 1984.

Offen, Karen. "Depopulation, Nationalism, and Feminism in Fin-de-Siècle France." *American Historical Review* 89, no. 3 (1984): 648–76.

Orbach, S. *Fat Is a Feminist Issue.* London: Arrow, 1978.

Pagès-Delon, Michèle. *Le corps et ses apparences: L'envers du look.* Paris: Éditions L'Harmattan, 1989.

Paquet, Dominique. *Miroir mon beau miroir: Une histoire de la beauté.* Paris: Gallimard, 1997.

Parkins, Ilya. *Poiret, Dior and Schiaparelli: Fashion, Femininity and Modernity.* New York, Berg, 2012.

Parkins, Wendy. "Moving Dangerously: Mobility and the Modern Woman." *Tulsa Studies in Women's Literature* 20, no. 1 (Spring 2001): 77–92.

Pateman, Carole. *The Sexual Contract.* Stanford, Calif.: Stanford University Press, 1988.

Peiss, Kathy. *Hope in a Jar: The Making of America's Beauty Culture.* New York: Henry Holt, 1998.

Perrot, Philippe. *Fashioning the Bourgeoisie: A History of Clothing in the Nineteenth Century.* Translated by Richard Bienvenu. Princeton, N.J.: Princeton University Press, 1994.

Pinset, Jacques, and Yvonne Deslandres. *Histoire des soins de beauté.* Paris: Presses Universitaires de France, 1960.

Plott, Michèle. "The Rules of the Game: Respectability, Sexuality, and the *Femme Mondaine* in Late-Nineteenth-Century Paris." *French Historical Studies* 25, no. 3 (Summer 2002): 531–56.

Pomfret, David. "'A Muse for the Masses': Gender, Age, and Nation in France, Fin de Siècle." *American Historical Review* 109, no. 4 (December 2004): 1439–74.

Poovey, Mary. *Uneven Developments: The Ideological Work of Gender in Mid-Victorian England.* Chicago: University of Chicago Press, 1988.

Pope, B. C. "The Influence of Rousseau's Ideology of Domesticity." In *Connecting Spheres: Women in the Western World 1500 to the Present,* edited by M. J. Boxer and J. H. Quataer. Oxford: Oxford University Press, 1987.

Rappaport, Erika Diane. *Shopping for Pleasure: Women in the Making of London's West End.* Princeton, N.J.: Princeton University Press, 2000.

Reynolds, Siân. *France between the Wars: Gender and Politics.* London: Routledge, 1996.

Roberts, Mary Louise. *Disruptive Acts: The New Woman in Fin-de-Siècle France.* Chicago: University of Chicago Press, 2002.

———. "Gender, Consumption and Commodity Culture." *American Historical Review* 103, no. 3 (June 1998): 817–44.

Roquilly, Christophe. *Le droit des produits cosmétiques.* Paris: Economica, 1991.

Rosenblatt, Helena. "On the "Misogyny" of Jean-Jacques Rousseau: The *Letter to d'Alembert* in Historical Context." *French Historical Studies* 25, no. 1 (Winter 2002): 91–114.

Ruffat, Michèle. "La recherche historique sur l'industrie pharmaceutique en France et à l'étranger." *Revue d'histoire de la pharmacie,* no. 305 (1995): 187–95.

———. *75 Years of French Pharmaceutical Industry: History of Synthélabo.* Paris: Éditions la découverte, 1996.

Saldern, Adelheid von. *The Challenge of Modernity: German Social and Cultural Studies, 1890–1960.* Ann Arbor: University of Michigan Press, 2002.

Schorske, Carl. *Fin de Siècle Vienna: Politics and Culture.* New York: Vintage, 1981.

Schwartz, Vanessa. *Spectacular Realities: Early Mass Culture in Fin-de-Siècle Paris.* Berkeley: University of California Press, 1999.

Scott, Joan. *The Fantasy of Feminist History.* Durham, N.C.: Duke University Press, 2011.

———. *Only Paradoxes to Offer: French Feminists and the Rights of Man.* Cambridge: Harvard University Press, 1996.

Silver, Kenneth E. "Purism: Straightening Up after the Great War." In *Modern Art and Society: An Anthology of Social and Multicultural Readings,* edited by Maurice Berger, 95–116. New York: Icon, 1994.

Silverman, Debora. "The 'New Woman,' Feminism, and the Decorative Arts in Fin-de-Siècle France." In *Eroticism and the Body Politic,* edited by Lynn Hunt, 144–63. Baltimore: Johns Hopkins University Press, 1991.

Smith, Bonnie. *Ladies of the Leisure Class: The Bourgeoises of Northern France in the Nineteenth Century.* Princeton, N.J.: Princeton University Press, 1981.

Sohn, Anne-Marie. "Between the Wars in France and England." In *Toward a Cultural Identity in the Twentieth Century,* edited by Françoise Thébaud, vol. 5 of *A History of Women in the West,* 92–119, Cambridge: Belknap Press of Harvard University Press, 1998.

———. "La garçonne face à l'opinion publique: Type littéraire ou type social des années 20?" *Le mouvement social,* no. 80 (July–September 1972): 3–27.

Solomon-Godeau, Abigail. "The Legs of the Countess." *October* 39 (Winter 1986): 65–108.

Steele, Valerie. *Fashion and Eroticism: Ideals of Feminine Beauty from the Victorian Era to the Jazz Age.* New York: Oxford University Press, 1985.

———. *Paris Fashion: A Cultural History.* New York: Oxford University Press 1988.

Stewart, Mary Lynn. *For Health and Beauty: Physical Culture for Frenchwomen, 1880s–1930s.* Baltimore: Johns Hopkins University Press, 2001.

Stora-Lamarre, Annie. *L'enfer de la IIIe République: Censeurs et pornographes, 1881–1914*. Paris: Imago, 1990.

Strasser, Susan, Charles McGovern, and Matthias Judt, eds. *Getting and Spending: European and American Consumer Societies in the Twentieth Century*. New York: Cambridge University Press, 1998.

Susman, Warren I. *Culture as History: The Transformation of American Society in the Twentieth Century*. New York: Pantheon, 1984.

Teal, Laurie. "The Hollow Women: Modernism, the Prostitute, and Commodity Aesthetics." *Differences* 7, no. 3 (Fall 1995): 80–108.

Thébaud, Françoise. "The Great War and the Triumph of Sexual Division." In *Toward a Cultural Identity in the Twentieth Century*, edited by Thébaud, vol. 5 of *A History of Women in the West*, 21–75. Cambridge: Belknap Press of Harvard University Press, 1998.

Thompson, Jan. "The Role of Women in the Iconography of Art Nouveau." *Art Journal* 31, no. 2 (Winter 1971–72): 158–67.

Thompson, Victoria. *The Virtuous Marketplace: Women and Men, Money and Politics, in Paris 1830–1870*. Baltimore: Johns Hopkins University Press, 2000.

Thurman, Judith. *Secrets of the Flesh: A Life of Colette*. New York: Knopf, 1999.

Tiersten, Lisa. *Marianne in the Market: Envisioning Consumer Society in Fin-de-Siècle France*. Berkeley: University of California Press, 2001.

Tilburg, Patricia. *Colette's Republic: Work, Gender, and Popular Culture in France, 1870–1914*. New York: Berghahn, 2009.

——. "Earning Her Bread: Métier, Order, and Female Honor in Colette's Music Hall, 1906–1913." *French Historical Studies* 28, no. 3 (Summer 2005): 497–530.

Troy, Nancy J. *Couture Culture: A Study of Modern Art and Fashion*. Cambridge: MIT Press, 2003.

Veblen, Thorstein. *Theory of the Leisure Class*. London: Sage, 1970.

Vigarello, Georges. *Concepts of Cleanliness: Changing Attitudes in France since the Middle Ages*. Translated by Jean Birrell. Cambridge: Cambridge University Press, 1988.

——. *Histoire de la beauté: Le corps et l'art d'embellir de la Renaissance à nos jours*. Paris: Hachette, 2004.

Weber, Eugen. *France: Fin de Siècle*. Cambridge: Belknap Press of Harvard University Press, 1986.

Weingarten, Rachel. *Hello Gorgeous! Beauty Products in America; '40s–'60s*. Portland, Ore.: Collector's Press, 2006.

Williams, Rosalind H. *Dream Worlds: Mass Consumption in Late Nineteenth-Century France*. Berkeley: University of California Press, 1982.

Wilson, Elizabeth. *Adorned in Dreams: Fashion and Modernity*. London: Virago, 1987.

Wolf, Naomi. *The Beauty Myth: How Images of Beauty Are Used Against Women*. New York: William Morrow, 1991

Woodhead, Lindy. *War Paint: Madame Helena Rubinstein and Miss Elizabeth Arden: Their Lives, Their Times, Their Rivalry*. Hoboken, N.J.: Wiley, 2003.

Zdatny, Steven. *Fashion, Work, and Politics in Modern France*. Palgrave Macmillan, 2006.

———. *Hairstyles and Fashion: A Hairdresser's History of Paris, 1910–1920*. New York: Bloomsbury Academic, 1999.

Index